TOTAL KNEE REPLACEMENT

12 Weeks to Success

Lori Marshall

Copyright © 2016 Lori Marshall
All rights reserved. This book or any portion thereof may not be reproduced or used in any manner whatsoever without the express written permission of the publisher except for the use of brief quotations in a book review.

www.thetotalkneereplacement.com

ISBN: 1535480920
ISBN-13: 978-1535480925

DEDICATION

For my patients, who provide me with so much professional joy, satisfaction and life lessons each and every day.

For Dr Mark Dekkers, Belinda and Rebecca for your professional and practical support over the past 6 years.

For my parents, who provide constant guidance, support and love to help me achieve my dreams.

For my husband, Evan and beautiful boys, Charlie and Henry - you are my dreams fulfilled! You constantly inspire me to reach higher, dig deeper and give more. I love you all so much.

> Thank you, all, for moulding me into the person I am today.
> I would be lost without you.

CONTENTS

    It's time   9
    What is a Total Knee Replacement?

1 Preparing for Surgery   13
        Preparation is Key
        Things to tell your Surgeon
        Questions to ask your Surgeon
        Risks & Complications
        General Risks of Surgery
        Total Knee Replacement Specific Risks
        Preparing yourself Mentally
        The Importance of a Support Network
        Sleep
        A word on Bilateral Knee Replacement
        All about Driving
        When can I Return to Work?
        When can I Return to Sport?
        When can I Return to Sex?
        Coping with Daily Activities
        Hospital Packing List

2 The Surgery   49
        Explaining the Procedure
        Medication
        Getting In & Out of Bed
        Using Crutches
        From Day 0 - Discharge

3 Your Exercise Program Explained   65
        Why Your Exercise Program is Important
        Key Points Before You Start...
        Types of Exercises

4 Exercises and Expectations from Discharge to 12   73
   Weeks & beyond
        Expectations Discharge - Week 2
        Exercises Week 1
        Exercises Week 2
        Expectations Weeks 2 - 4

        Exercises Week 3
        Exercises Week 4
        Expectations Weeks 4 - 6
        Exercises Week 5
        Exercises Week 6
        Expectations Weeks 6 - 8
        Exercises Week 6 - 8
        Expectations Weeks 8 - 12
        Exercises Week 8 - 10
        Exercises Week 10 - 12
        Expectations Week 12 and beyond
        Exercises Week 12 and beyond...
        It's up to you...

5   Glossary   134

6   Bibliography   136

Disclaimer

The information provided in this book is designed to provide helpful information on Total Knee Replacements, and should not be construed as personal medical advice. This book is not meant to be used, nor should it be used, to diagnose or treat any medical condition. You have not become a patient of Lori Marshall by reading these pages, and you should consult with your personal physician/care giver regarding your own medical care. For diagnosis or treatment of any medical problem, please consult your own physician. Lori Marshall is not responsible for any specific health or allergy needs that may require medical supervision and is not liable for any damages or negative consequences from any treatment, action, application or preparation, to any person reading or following the information in this book. As with any new exercise program, you should consult your doctor for approval prior to commencement. If, while exercising, you feel unwell, dizzy, short of breath or feel chest pain, please speak with your doctor. References are provided for informational purposes only and do not constitute endorsement of any websites or other sources. Readers should be aware that the websites listed in this book may change.

It's time

Your knee hurts. A lot. All the time.

It feels stiff and sore when you wake in the morning. So you limp to the medicine cabinet and pop a few pain relievers whilst heating up a hot pack and strapping on your knee support. It's stopping you from enjoying your life, and you've had enough.

So you speak to your doctor about it.

What? A knee replacement? No, I don't need a knee replacement. Isn't it risky? My brother's total knee replacement didn't go so well. I'm not so sure…

Guess what?

Total knee replacements can give you back the life you deserve.

Follow my 12 week plan and feel confident that you will get the most out of your new knee. You are investing a lot of time, money and a little discomfort in your new knee. You owe it to yourself to complete a clear, graduated exercise program that will have you feeling fantastic in only 12 weeks.

Learn how to help yourself before the surgery to fast track your recovery.
Know, in advance, what to expect week by week.

Most importantly, recover with confidence, knowing that you are giving your new knee the best possible chance to reach its full potential.

How to use this book

Do not read this book cover to cover. Instead, I recommend you read the section that applies to you at the time. So if you are preparing for surgery, you should be reading the Preparing For Surgery section. Equally, if you are newly discharged from hospital, go straight to the section Exercises and Expectations From Discharge to 12 Weeks and Beyond.

Bonus Exercise Planner!
If you would like a free 12 Week Exercise Planner to help keep track of your exercises, visit www.thetotalkneereplacement.com and enter your name and email address and you will receive a printable PDF in your in-box.

Together, we can help your new knee achieve its full potential.

Now let's get started...

What is a Total Knee Replacement?

What is it?

A Total Knee Replacement is a major surgical procedure, where the damaged areas of the knee joint are replaced with a metal and plastic artificial knee joint. It is also known as a "Knee Arthroplasty".

Why do you need one?

The Australian Orthopaedic Association (AOA) states that Total Knee Replacements may be recommended for people with:
- Chronic pain that has not been relieved by anti-inflammatory medications, physiotherapy, and the use of a walking stick or other devices.
- Severe knee pain that restricts work, walking, recreation and daily activities.
- Disturbed sleep due to night pain.
- A very stiff knee that is possibly swollen.
- Advanced arthritis confirmed by x-ray.
- Avascular necrosis (lack of blood supply) which has damaged the knee joint, usually caused by trauma.

Can I avoid having one?

Some people find that pursuing a weight loss and supervised strengthening and exercise program actually reduces their knee pain to the point that a knee replacement is no longer required. The use of knee supports and a walking stick may also extend the life of your natural knee. Your surgeon will remind you, however, that these options do not change the arthritis in your knee, and that later on you may still require surgery to remove the arthritic joint. However, they are worthwhile options to pursue, especially if you are under the age of 70.

How long do they last?

Approximately 25 years, but this is improving all the time. This is why we wait until you are older if possible. Knee replacements also last longer in people who are of lighter weight.

Can anyone have a Total Knee Replacement?

No.
According to the AOA, your surgeon will usually not recommend a Total Knee Replacement for people who have:
- Severe obesity
- Severe Peripheral Vascular Disease
- An infection in the knee or leg
- A nerve disorder affecting the knee
- Severe, uncontrolled Parkinson's Disease

This is due to the high risk of failure of the prosthesis in patients with these conditions.

You will also be assessed for your suitability for the anaesthetic drugs. Significant heart and lung disease may put you at greater risk of complications from a general anaesthetic. You may be able to use a different type of anaesthetic during surgery, but this will be up to your surgeon and anaesthetist.

1

Preparing for Surgery

Preparation is Key

In the weeks leading up to your surgery, there are plenty of things to consider that make the first few weeks after surgery a little easier…

Home help
If you usually live alone, arrange to have someone stay with you at home for your first 2 – 3 weeks after surgery. You will be sore, tired and the medication can make you feel a bit cloudy in the head. Prepare and freeze meals in advance. Do not stress about the housework!! The dusting, vacuuming, weeding, gardening and ironing can wait. If it is going to bother you, try to have it all up to date prior to surgery and have a friend, family member or local service keep things going whilst you are unable.

Medications
Ensure you have told your surgeon about **ALL** the tablets/medication you take – even over the counter things like vitamins and supplements. These can have a real impact on the drugs you are given in hospital. Things such as iron tablets, fish oil or glucosamine supplements can affect how much bleeding you'll have after surgery. Write a list down and give it to your doctor at least a fortnight in advance.

Smoking
You should stop smoking at least a fortnight prior to your surgery. Smoking increases the risk of a poor outcome after surgery as it impairs healing.

Dentistry
You will need to arrange any urgent or necessary dental work to be completed prior to your knee replacement. After your knee surgery, inform your dentist about your new knee, as you will need to take antibiotics prior to each visit to the dentist for the next 2 years. Yes, this includes simple dental check-ups.

Equipment

Arrange to have the appropriate equipment in your home ready on the day you are discharged from hospital.

You **will** need:

- *Over toilet frame:* This raises the toilet seat higher to make it easier to get on/off. You will need this for approximately 6 weeks.

- *Crutches:* 6 weeks

- *Bed:* Just for yourself for the first few weeks. It will be much more comfortable for both you and your spouse. Make sure your bed is not too low, such as a futon or (gasp!) a water bed. Beds that are too low make it too difficult to get up.

- *Chair:* This must be a high firm chair to make it easier for you to get in/out of it. The seat needs to be slightly higher than the distance from the floor to your knee. Up to 6 weeks.

- *Roll towel:* Get your biggest/thickest towel. Hold the towel vertically, and then fold it in half length ways. Roll it up so it looks like a log. This needs to be a thick roll, similar to a paint tin. If it is too thin, incorporate a second towel. Use tape or rubber bands to secure it in place.

- *Skateboard:* Don't stress, I'll tell you more about this further down the page!

- *Ice packs:* You'll need these for the first few weeks in particular. These need to be bendable. A hard ice brick won't work well.

- *Shower Chair:* A non-wheeled sturdy plastic chair for your shower. It must have non-slip feet and slots for the water to drain through.

- *Non-slip shower mat:* To ensure that you don't slip over on the slippery, sudsy shower floor.

You **may** also need:
- *Bath Board:* If your shower is over the bath
- *Long handled Shoe horn:* To help put on slip-on shoes
- *Sock donner:* To help put on socks
- *Easy-Reacher/Pickup stick:* To help pick things up off the floor. A long handled pair of tongs would also work well.

Pre-Surgical Exercises
Performing some basic strengthening exercises prior to your surgery will make the first few weeks after surgery less difficult. Position yourself face up on your bed. Do these exercises on BOTH legs.

You should perform the following exercises 3 x a day, **every day** prior to surgery:

1. *Ankle pumps:* Bend your ankles up and down to reduce ankle stiffness and improve circulation. Perform 20 ankle pumps.

2. *Thigh squeezes:* Try to straighten your knee by squeezing your thigh muscles (your Quadriceps muscle). Visualise your knee cap moving towards your hip. Press your heel away from you. Hold the squeeze for 3 seconds. Repeat this 10 times each leg.

3. *Inner Range Quads:* Place your Roll Towel under your knee. Slowly straighten your knee and hold it for 3 seconds, then lower it back to the bed. Repeat this 10 times per leg.

4. *Straight Leg Raise:* Perform a Thigh Squeeze (above) and slowly lift your leg up 30 cm above the bed, <u>keeping your knee perfectly straight</u>. Then, slowly lower it back down to the bed. Remember – the point is to keep your knee locked straight. So don't allow your knee to sag, either on the way up or down. The height you lift it up does NOT matter! Perform this 10 times on each leg.

5. *Heel slides:* Slide your heel towards your bottom and then straighten it back out again. Perform this 10 times on each leg.

Physiotherapy

You should arrange to have a physiotherapist see you once you are home from hospital. You can choose to see your local physiotherapist in their clinic, or source a physiotherapist that does home visits. As a guide, they should see you weekly until 4 weeks, then fortnightly until 8 - 10 weeks, although this may vary patient to patient. Bilateral knee replacements should be seen 1 - 2 x weekly until 6 weeks, weekly until 8 - 10 weeks and then fortnightly if required, due to the extra time needed to manage both replacements properly.
Check with your health insurer to find out your level of cover for physiotherapy services. You can obtain the relevant health insurance item numbers from your physiotherapist at the time of booking.

Weight

As you get heavier, your knee needs to cope with more and more force every single step you take. Excess weight can magnify the effects of arthritis on your knee joint and cause more pain and joint inflammation. Equally, after surgery, excess weight can increase the rate of wear and tear on your new knee and contribute to increased pain during the rehab process. If at all possible, try to reduce your body weight in the lead up to your surgery by eating a nutritious, balanced diet and increasing your level of exercise. Low impact exercise such as swimming and cycling can increase your metabolism without straining your sore knee.

Pre-operative tests

You will have a blood test, ECG and a chest x-ray approximately 1 week prior to your surgery. You will need to refrain from gardening, mowing the lawn or any other activity that may result in a scratch, cut or bite to your leg. Any breakage of your skin may result in your surgery being cancelled due to the increased risk of infection. Be sure to notify your surgeon in the event that a cut, scratch or bite occurs in the week leading up to your surgery.

Consent Form

Once you have agreed to surgery, you will be asked to sign a consent form. Please read this carefully and ask your surgeon any questions you may have before signing it.

Things to tell your Surgeon

Prior to surgery
You should tell your Surgeon about:
- How your knee affects your activities of daily living
- Your full medical history, in particular:
    - Previous knee surgery and how you recovered
    - Previous clots
    - Excessive bleeding or bruising
    - Heart problems
    - Lung problems or breathing difficulties
    - Psychological or psychiatric illnesses
    - Gout
    - Diabetes
    - History of keloid scars or poor healing of scars after previous surgery
- Allergies or previous bad reactions to anaesthetics, surgical tape, wound dressings, antibiotics and other medications
- Whether you have a support network at home after surgery
- All medications you take - prescribed and over the counter
- All vitamins, minerals and supplements you are taking
- Any cuts, bites or scratches to your legs that occur in the week prior to surgery
- Any concerns or worries you may have about the surgery

After surgery
Please inform your surgery if any of the following occur:
- Body temperature of greater than 38.5°C/101°F
- Shaking chills
- Severe pain or tenderness during activity and at rest
- Heavy bleeding from the incisions
- Redness around the incision that is spreading
- Nausea or vomiting
- Decreasing ability to bend your knee
- A fall that results in reduced mobility
- Any concerns you may have

Questions to ask your Surgeon

Most surgeons and hospitals will have their own booklets with information on your anaesthetic, wound care, pain relief options, basic exercises etc. However, it is wise to write down a list of questions to take with you to your surgeon to ask prior to surgery. Research shows that most patients only retain 35% of what they are told during a consultation with a doctor. Take a support person with you to be a "second set of ears".

Can you please explain the procedure?
You should be provided an outline of what will happen during surgery. How long it takes, the name/type of prosthesis and how it is fitted to your knee joint.

What type of anaesthetic will be used? Any risks or side effects?
You may be directed to your anaesthetist's office for further information.

What is your complication rate? What types of complications?
How many times do things go wrong per 100 surgeries? A list of things to monitor in the post-surgical period.

What is the failure rate of the prosthesis that you use? Why do you use that particular one?
You can learn about your new knee and potential issues to monitor.

How long will I be in hospital?
Usually 4 - 7 days depending on your individual medical history.

Will I need to go to a extended stay rehabilitation unit?
This is a decision between you and your surgeon and depends on your support network at home. If you are really worried about how you will cope in the first few weeks after surgery, this can be an important discussion.

What are the item numbers for the surgery and the anaesthetist, the total cost, and the out of pocket cost?
This is so that you can contact your health fund to confirm your out of pocket charges prior to surgery.

When can I drive again?
Usually 6 weeks, but it is good to confirm this with your surgeon and your car insurance cover.

How long should I wear the compression stockings?
Usually for 6 weeks.

What are my pain relief options and what should I do if I require further scripts?
Talk about the pain medication regime, common side effects and generally how long you are expected to take them. Double check that there are no expected interactions with any of your regular medications that you may take for other health conditions.

What should I look for with blood clots and what should I do in the event that I suspect one, both during the week and on the weekend?
Your surgeon should outline the common signs of a blood clot and whether to call their office or go straight to the hospital's Emergency Department.

What should I look for with wound infection and what should I do in the event that I suspect my wound is infected - during the week and on the weekend?
Your surgeon should outline the common signs of an infection and whether to call their office, see your family doctor or go straight to the Emergency Department.

What are my goals for my 6 week review and my 12 week review?
This will help you monitor your progress, but remember - everyone is different!

When do you think I will return to work?
If you need to return to work - so you can let your workplace know.

Can I return to my sport? How long until I can return to my sport?
If you wish to return to sport - is your sport appropriate for knee replacements? Ask for a list of approved sports.

Do you have a recommendation for a physiotherapist? Can they come to my house?
Your surgeon may have a preferred physiotherapist, or they may be happy for you to see your local therapist.

How long should the wound remain covered?
This is important for prevention of infection.

What should I do if one of the dissolvable stitches doesn't seem to have dissolved? How long should I wait?
This question can be held off until after surgery. It will help you monitor your wound.

Risks & Complications

Listed below are the risks and complications you should be monitoring…

General risks of Surgery
- Pain
- Nausea
- Allergies
- Damage to nerves and blood vessels
- Heavy bleeding
- Scarring

Specific risks for Total Knee Replacement
- Infection
- Blood clots
- Loosening of prosthesis
- Breakage of prosthesis
- Dislocation of the new knee joint
- Bone fracture around the prosthesis
- Stiffness
- Severely impaired blood supply
- Drainage of fluid build up
- Numbness of the skin around the wound
- Revision
- Adhesions

General Risks of Surgery

Let's look at the general risks of surgery a little more closely...

Pain
You may feel pain:
- around the incision site, and where the drain was inserted;
- due to the application of a tourniquet during surgery above and below your knee;
- due to the swelling around your new knee;
- on moving your new knee for the first few weeks;
- for the first few months.

You will be provided pain relief medication to address your pain. If you have any concerns, please speak with your surgeon.

Nausea
You may feel nausea in the period after surgery due to the anaesthesia and pain relief medications. This usually settles quickly, but speak with your surgeon if you are concerned by its ongoing nature.

Allergies
You may suffer from an allergy to:
- the anaesthetic drugs;
- the pain relief medication;
- the antiseptic solutions used on your skin;
- the medical stitches;
- the wound dressings or the medical tape.

Speak with your surgeon or practice nurse regarding any allergies you may encounter.

Damage to the nerves and blood vessels
You may incur damage to both major and minor nerves and blood vessels from the surgical procedure. This injury may be temporary or permanent. Nerve damage can lead to poor or no muscle strength in your leg. Most minor nerve injuries repair over time. If you are still

unable to straighten your knee, or perform a straight leg raise by Week 3 - speak with your surgeon.

Heavy Bleeding

You may experience heavy bleeding from the surgical site which may require a blood transfusion. It is important that you notify your surgeon prior to surgery regarding any previous history of excessive bleeding and bruising. You should have also discussed any medical conditions that cause you to bleed excessively, as well as any medications and supplements you are taking that may increase your risk of excessive bleeding.

Scarring

You may develop keloid scarring along your incision. This is where the scar remains raised, thick, itchy and red. Keloid scars are not dangerous to your health, but they may be annoying and be a cosmetic concern.

Total Knee Replacement Specific Risks

Now let's look at the risks specific to total knee replacements…

1. Infection
Infection can spread from any part of your body to your new knee. Most common points of entry for bacteria into the bloodstream include from dental work, urinary tract infections and skin infections. Bacteria can also enter through the incision itself.

Whilst the risk of infection around the prosthesis is roughly 1 in 100, it must be taken very seriously. At worst, if the bacteria is resistant to antibiotics, it can lead to further surgery to remove your new knee joint.

Warning Signs of Infection
- Body temperature greater than 38.5°C/101°F
- Shaking chills
- Redness around the incision that is spreading
- Decreasing ability to bend your knee
- Drainage of pus or fluid from your wound
- Increasing knee pain both during activity and at rest

What to do
Report any warning signs to your Surgeon immediately. You will be given antibiotics and monitored closely.

How to avoid Infections
- Keep the wound is covered for roughly 2 - 3 weeks
- Once the wound is uncovered, avoid touching the wound areas that are not fully closed
- Arrange to have any necessary dental procedures done prior to your knee surgery
- Avoid swimming pools until the wound is fully closed (scabs have fallen off and just a scar remains)

An Important note on Dentists
After your surgery, you will need to inform your Dentist or Orthodontist prior to each visit. You are encouraged to avoid dental work for at least the first three months after surgery unless absolutely necessary. You will need to take preventative antibiotics before and after each visit for at least the first 2 years after surgery. This is to reduce the risk of bacteria entering your bloodstream in your mouth and causing an infection around your prosthesis.

2. Blood Clots

You are most at risk of developing a blood clot during the first few weeks of your recovery.
You will need to wear a pair of compression stockings as directed by your surgeon - usually for the first 6 weeks. You will also be on blood thinning medication for approximately 10 days after surgery. You must be particularly watchful if you have had prior clots.

Warning signs of Blood Clots
- Increasing pain or tenderness in calf muscle or behind the knee
- Increased swelling in the calf, ankle and foot
- Redness above or below the knee

What to do
Call your Surgeon's office and report it immediately. They will advise whether you need to go in and see them, obtain an ultrasound, or go straight to the Emergency Department.

How to avoid Blood Clots
- Wear your compression stockings on both legs for the first 6 weeks except when you are showering
- Ensure that there are no creases in the stockings while you wear them
- Take your blood thinning medication as directed by your Surgeon

- Ensure you report any history of blood clots to your Surgeon prior to surgery
- Perform your circulatory exercises - Foot/Ankle pumps, thigh squeezes and buttock squeezes hourly for the first week, and then 3 x day until 6 weeks.
- Attempt to mobilise regularly throughout the day
- Change your position regularly

3. Pulmonary Embolisms

Pulmonary Embolisms are Blood Clots that have dislodged from your deep leg veins and travelled to your lungs.

Warning signs of a Pulmonary Embolism
- Sudden shortness of breath
- Sudden sharp chest pain which may increase with coughing or deep breathing
- Coughing up blood
- Fainting
- Rapid pulse or irregular heartbeat
- Anxiety or sweating

What to do
*Call an ambulance immediately and follow the operator's instructions **- this is a medical emergency***

How to avoid Pulmonary Embolisms
- Report all symptoms of a Blood Clot to your Surgeon immediately.
- Follow the advice for the prevention of Blood Clots.

4. Revisions

A revision is a procedure where the prosthesis in your new knee is removed and replaced with another one. These occur due to loosening of the replacement; infection surrounding your new knee joint; or a fall causing a breakage of the prosthesis or the surrounding bone. A revision may also occur in a patient who received a knee replacement at a relatively young age, and the replacement has reached the end of its lifespan.

Revisions don't rehabilitate as well as the initial replacement as there is less bone stock to hold the prosthesis and the range achieved is usually less. This is why you must look after your new knee carefully.

5. Stiffness

Stiffness is both a short term and long term complication. You will feel knee stiffness for the first few weeks due to pain and swelling. However, without proper exercise and movement, the stiffness can carry on to become a long term complication and affect your ability to perform your regular activities, such as putting on sneakers and walking up stairs. If your knee was particularly stiff prior to surgery, you may still suffer from ongoing stiffness afterward.

6. Drainage of Fluid

You may experience a build-up of fluid in the knee joint which may not reabsorb naturally, and so may require drainage.

7. Severely impaired blood supply

In the rare event (1 in 6000) of complications from the surgery causing severely impaired blood supply to the leg, the leg may need amputation. This risk is greater with increasing age or poor health. Your surgeon will screen for these risk factors prior to recommending surgery, thus greatly reducing the risk of this complication.

8. Numbness

You may feel numbness around the area of the wound. This is due to the smaller nerves in the skin being cut during surgery. This numbness of the skin reduces over time as the nerves regenerate.

9. Adhesions

Adhesions are thick, heavy scar tissues that prevent the structures in and around your knee from gliding over each other and restricts the bending of your knee. They occur in roughly 4% of total knee replacements. You may need to undergo a "Manipulation under Anaesthesia" to release the tight scar tissues and improve your range of movement. This is why it is important to perform your exercise program moderately and regularly.

Those who don't move their knee enough, due to pain or non-compliance, can develop adhesions.
Those who undergo hyper-aggressive physiotherapy or overdo their exercise program can also develop adhesions.

Equally, there are some patients who do everything as directed and still develop adhesions.

10. Manipulation Under Anaesthesia

Manipulation Under Anaesthesia (MUA) may be required if your new knee remains very stiff despite physiotherapy and regular exercise past Week 10. If, by this time, your new knee is still not bending past 100 degrees, your surgeon will consider a MUA. It is a non-surgical procedure where you are put under a general or spinal anaesthetic to allow your surgeon to move your knee in order to break any adhesions that are restricting your movement.

Your surgeon can freely bend and straighten your knee during the procedure as the anaesthetic completely blocks the sensation of pain and relaxes any muscle contractions. They will move your knee joint and be able to feel where the adhesions are blocking further gains in range of movement. Your surgeon will perform specific manoeuvres in order to tear the adhesions and achieve full range of movement.

This can be performed as a day procedure, but many surgeons have their patients admitted for a couple of days for twice daily physiotherapy treatment and use of a Continuous Passive Motion (CPM) machine after the MUA. This ensures the newly gained range is maintained and the adhesions do not reform.

Risks
Like all procedures, a MUA carries risks related to the use of anaesthesia, as well as the possibility that the force needed to break the thick adhesions, may cause a bony fracture. As such, surgeons may avoid performing a MUA on patients with osteoporosis, or patients who carry higher than normal risks with anaesthetic due to their age, or those suffering from a heart or lung condition.

An MUA is not a failure or an indication of lack of compliance. I have seen patients need a MUA due to their poor compliance with their exercise plan due to pain or lack of motivation. But I have also seen a MUA required despite rigorous compliance with the exercise program.

The window of opportunity for a MUA appears to be from Week 10 until Week 16. Often poor range will be noted at the Week 6 appointment and reviewed at Week 12. If your bend has not improved sufficiently, you may be advised to undergo a MUA.

Fear of MUA
Many patients refuse a MUA due to their fear of having to undergo further hospitalisation, anaesthetic or pain. It is important to note that this is a procedure and not surgery. You are not "opened up" again. The anaesthetic is simply to block the sensation of pain you would

otherwise feel as the adhesions are being broken. The procedure itself only takes a few minutes. The results can really be astonishing and the short term impact of a few days in hospital and a slight short term increase in pain and swelling is completely outweighed by the benefit of an extra 10 - 30 degrees of knee bend every day for the rest of your life!

Preparing yourself Mentally

Recovery from total knee replacement is just as much a mental battle as it is a physical one.

You will have good days and bad days.

Good hours and bad hours.

This up and down journey will continue for at least the first few months in some way.

My knee will be fixed today

The main problem for many patients is that they have circled the date of the surgery on their calendar and think to themselves…
"This is the day my knee will finally feel better!"
They may even have a star or a smiley face next to it.

The trouble with this scenario is, your knee will not feel that much better initially. So it can feel very disappointing when you have visualised a pain free knee on a certain date, to wake up 4 weeks later after broken sleep with a knee that is still sore, slightly swollen and somewhat stiff. In fact, it is extremely common around the 3 - 4 week mark to feel quite angry, frustrated, teary and worried that perhaps the surgery wasn't successful. In all likelihood, your knee is totally fine and progressing well. It's just different to your expectations. Many patients feel their second knee replacement is much easier than their first. This is mostly due to a better alignment of expectations with reality.

Another source of frustration is comparing yourself with your spouse, neighbour, another patient in the waiting room, or golfing buddy. Please don't! Everyone's history and personal circumstances are different. It is not a competition or a race. You should be focused on achieving your goals through to 12 weeks and beyond, to 12 months.

Travel the middle road

Generally speaking, the outcomes at 12 weeks after surgery are better for people who approach their TKR rehab with **moderation and patience**.

Those who are lazy and do not perform their exercises as directed have bad outcomes at 12 weeks and 12 months - a stiff, painful knee that doesn't bend or straighten fully. These patients often ask, "What is the minimum amount of exercise required?" or they may skip exercise sessions altogether, citing pain or fatigue. *If this sounds familiar, your physiotherapist will need to kick you into gear.*

Equally, those who push too hard have bad outcomes at 12 weeks. These are the patients who do 30 repetitions of each exercise when they are told to do 10. Or they may walk for 45 minutes, when they are instructed to walk for 20 minutes.
These patients may seem ahead of the pack around 6 weeks, but overdoing it leads to increased swelling and pain, stiffening of the knee and loss of movement. *If this sounds familiar, your physiotherapist will need to put the reins on you.*

Please simply follow the instructions from this book and your physiotherapist to improve slowly but surely.

A is for Attitude

Your recovery is determined by the skill of your surgeon, your condition prior to surgery and your attitude.

A positive attitude where you take responsibility for your recovery will help enormously. Ensure you have enough sedate interests such as reading, movies, handiwork, crosswords and the like to provide pleasant distraction through the first few weeks. Gradually increase how much you help around the house and see the rehabilitation period as a chance to catch up on some rest, a new novel, or the latest series of your favourite television show.

A negative attitude can lead to a poor recovery

The following thoughts or attitudes are not helpful:

- Thinking the worst: *"My knee feels painful - there must be something wrong with it."*
- Finding painful experiences unbearable: *The reaction to pain is greater than the pain itself.*
- Regret: *"I should never have had my knee replaced."*
- Over-reliance on pain medication for a long period: *"I just can't cope without them."*
- Being overly focused on your recovery: *This can lead to becoming overly anxious and distressed.*
- Worrying about returning to work: *"If I go back to work my pain will get worse."*
- Fear of movement and exercise because the knee is swollen or hurts.
- Not taking responsibility for your actions or contribution to your recovery: *Expecting your surgeon, physiotherapist or GP to solve all your problems.*
- Financial issues or concerns with insurance claims.
- Negative attitudes or unhelpful beliefs from your support network.
- Misunderstandings between you and your doctor or physiotherapist.
- Social isolation and becoming disconnected from the community.

Have a read through the list above. Can you see yourself in there?

If the answer is YES, make an appointment to see your doctor to talk through your concerns. Get on top of your feelings now so that you can move forwards with your recovery.

The Importance of a Supportive Network

Patients who have a supportive Spouse/Family/Friend/Caregiver typically recover faster than those who go home alone.

Your support network can help you with:

- Household tasks such as cooking, cleaning, laundry, ironing, gardening and shopping.
- Care needs such as getting compression stockings on and off or being there "just in case" at shower time.
- Driving to and from appointments and taking you out and about once you feel up to it.
- Providing comfort, support and a cup of tea when you feel tired, emotional, cranky, teary, frustrated or are in pain.
- Gently reminding you to do your exercises, take your medicine, eat a healthy diet and get enough rest.

Your support network will have their work cut out for them over the first few weeks.
Go give them a hug right now!

What to do if you are on your own

If you do not have a support network who can help you for the first 2 - 3 weeks, there are some things you can do prior to surgery to make the initial rehab period easier:

- You will need to arrange for someone to drive you home from hospital on the day of discharge.
- Consider arranging a carer to help you for the first 2 weeks.
- Arrange the equipment you will need in advance.
- Prepare and freeze your meals for the first 2 weeks in advance. Eating a healthy diet promotes healing and gives you energy for the rehab period.
- If your bedroom is upstairs, arrange to sleep downstairs for the first 2-3 weeks.

- Ensure there are clear, open pathways from your bed to the bathroom, and through the living areas so that you can use your crutches or walker safely.
- Remove any rugs, mat, power cords and phone cords to avoid any trips or falls.
- Ensure you have a light switch or lamp next to your bed in case you need to get up at night time.
- Do your grocery shopping ahead of time, shop for groceries on-line, or arrange delivery of your groceries for the first 3 - 4 weeks.
- Place all the items you use often, such as phone, remote control, medications, water bottle, tissues or a book within easy reach of your bed and chair. You may wish to use a back pack or other bag to carry them from room to room.

You can still reach your knee's full potential with a bit of planning and forward thinking.

Sleep

Getting a good night sleep is very important! Unfortunately, for the first few weeks after a knee replacement, your sleep overnight will be broken. This will be due to breakthrough pain and difficulties finding a comfortable position to spend the night.

Sleep positions
For the first 4 - 6 weeks, you will need to be sleeping on your back. This may be challenging for those more accustomed to sleeping on their sides, or heaven forbid, on their stomachs! It will also affect those who sleep on their sides to avoid snoring. Please do not place a pillow underneath your knee, as this encourages your knee to remain slightly bent, and may reduce your chances of achieving full knee extension. You do not need to sleep overnight with your leg elevated on pillows unless your leg is especially swollen. Instead, elevate your leg when resting during the afternoon.

Sleep and Pain relief
Pain feels worse when you are tired and have a poor night's sleep. It is important that you continue to take your pain relief to limit overnight pain so that you can enjoy better quality sleep. In the early weeks after surgery, it is important to rest, or even nap, in the afternoon to offset the effect of reduced sleep time overnight.

Sleep and Mental Health
It is lack of sleep that significantly contributes to patients feeling teary, frustrated and emotional around weeks 2 - 4. You are simply exhausted from the lack of sleep! Understanding that interrupted sleep, whilst incredibly frustrating, is quite normal for the first few weeks may help to ease the emotional stress you are feeling, as well as help your concerned spouse or support person to understand your emotions.

Sleep and your Partner
You will need to sleep in your own bed for the first few weeks. You may be restless overnight, and an accidental bump from your partner may not be as welcome as usual! It will also help your spouse or support person to get a good night sleep as they work extra hard to care

for you in those early weeks. If your bedroom is upstairs and living area is downstairs, it may be best to set up a bed downstairs for you to sleep in initially.

Sleep strategies

When you are waking through the night due to knee pain, you should take extra pain relief. You can also try doing your bed exercises - thigh squeezes, ankle pumps, bending your knee to your chest - to help ease the stiffness and reduce your pain. An ice pack applied to your knee for 20 minutes may also provide temporary pain relief and allow you to return to sleep. Depending on the season, some people find the winter covers too heavy on their knee. You can obtain a bed cradle which lifts the covers up off your leg, but still keeps you warm overnight.

A word on Bilateral Knee Replacements…

Having both knees replaced at the same time is a very tough. You may be in a position where you have no choice.

My strong advice to you is to obtain more than one opinion and, if possible, speak to someone who has experienced this type of surgery.

Sometimes it is easier to do your worse knee and then the other knee 12 weeks later.

Yes - this will lock you into a 6 month rehabilitation.
Yes - you may think "While I'm getting one done, I may as well get both done".

But if you undertake a bilateral knee replacement the reality is…
- You will be slower with your recovery by at least 2 - 3 weeks
- You may be in more pain as you have no "good leg" to rely upon
- You will find it a more difficult recovery

If you decide to go ahead with the bilateral knee replacement surgery, you will need to further adjust your expectations, and add 2 weeks onto each milestone.
You will require more patience and a longer period of pain relief.
You will definitely need a support network to help you for the first 6 weeks.
Read **Preparing yourself Mentally** and if you identify with the comments listed, think long and hard before agreeing to such surgery.

If you are comfortable and choose to go ahead - all the information contained in this book applies to you, too.

All about Driving

Getting in and out of the car after surgery can be daunting for some.

Getting into the car after surgery

The easiest way to get in and out of the car is:

- Position the front passenger seat as far back as possible.
- Open the car door wide and wind the window down.
- Approach the passenger side with your crutches and turn so that your back is facing the seat.
- Back up carefully until your legs can feel the car behind you.
- Give your crutches to the driver and hold onto the window sill and the car frame or the back of your seat for support.
- Position your operated leg a half step forward of your strong leg.
- *Bend your head and chest forward and stick your bottom backwards as you lower yourself towards the seat with your strong leg. **Watch your head!**
- Slide your bottom backwards so that you are securely on the seat.
- **Pivot so that you are facing the front of the car, lifting one leg in at a time.

*If you find that you are not getting your bottom securely on the seat, lean forward further as you sit down. This pushes your bottom back further so that it is closer to the middle of the seat.
**If you find the pivot to the front difficult because you are sticking to your seat, try placing a garbage bag on the seat before you sit down. The plastic sides of the bag slip on one another, making the pivot easier.

Getting out of the car

The procedure is the reverse:

- Open the door and wind the window down so that you can support yourself on the window sill.
- Have your driver bring your crutches around to your side so that they are there when you need them.
- Slowly pivot and lift one leg out of the car at a time.
- Slide your bottom forward towards the edge of the seat. This makes standing up easier.
- Position your operated leg a half step ahead of your strong leg.
- Hold onto the window sill and the frame of the car.
- Lean forward, pushing through your arms to stand up.
- Grab your crutches - and you're off!

When can I drive again?

This is often the first question patients ask their doctor or physiotherapist.

The answer is **around the 6 week mark**, after your surgeon has given you the all clear at your 6 week review appointment.

In fact, the Arthroplasty Society of Australia recommends not driving for a minimum period of six weeks following knee replacement surgery.

This is regardless of:

- Whether your left or right knee was replaced.
- Whether you drive a manual or automatic car.

The Slam the Brakes test

After this six week period, you can resume driving provided you feel confident to control the vehicle safely. I call this the "Slam the Brakes" test. You can resume driving once you are confident that you could, without hesitation, slam the brakes if a child or animal darted out on the road in front of you.

Insurance Issues

You also need to consider if there are any Car Insurance issues. As there are so many variations of insurance policies, it is very important that you check with your car's insurer prior to surgery. Your insurer may require you to wait until you have received the "all-clear" from your surgeon prior to covering you again. If you drive before receiving a doctor's clearance, or before the time the insurer indicates in their policy, you may not be covered if you are involved in a car accident, regardless of who was at fault!

When can I Return to Work?

If you are seeking to return to work, the time-frame for your return is really dependent on the type of work you do, and if there are light/appropriate duties that you can perform whilst you are still recovering. As a guide, office workers can return to work around weeks 6 - 8, whereas more physical workers such as nurses return to work around week 12. If you are a tradesman, it can be even later, into week 14, before you are back toward full work duties.

Remember, regardless of the type of work you do, you will have lost a lot of work fitness. You will feel extra tired during and after work for the first few weeks. You may need to consider if a graduated return to work is possible. For example, 2 days the first week, 3 days the second week, and full time from the third week. This may allow you to return to work sooner, albeit working fewer hours. You can also consider if working from home is a possibility to speed up your return.

One thing many people forget to consider is the commute to and from work. If you catch a bus or train to work, you need to ensure that you are confident with the distance to and from the station. It is recommended that you sit for the journey, rather than stand.

You should write down a list of all the tasks/duties you need to perform throughout the week, and make sure that you are strong enough to perform them, before you return to work. Can you practice these tasks in the fortnight leading up to your return to enable a smooth transition back to work?

When can I Return to Sport?

Sport is a part of many people's lives. Once you have had a total knee replacement, you are allowed to participate in:
- Walking
- Swimming
- Aqua Aerobics
- Golf
- Pilates
- Cycling/Exercise bike
- Bowls

You should return to sport in conjunction with your surgeon's advice. Discuss your desire to return to your chosen sport prior to surgery, and then again at your 6 week review. Your return date really depends on the type of sport you play.

Things you can do to improve your chances of returning to sport include:
- Keep your body weight down to reduce the load on your new knee
- Improve your general fitness with walking, hydrotherapy and exercise bike practice
- Continue your strength and balance exercise program well past the 12 week mark
- Commence Sport specific drills or part practice from week 6 - 8, depending on your sport and how you are feeling.

When can I Return to Sex?

The general advice for returning to sex is when you feel comfortable. This is often around the 4 - 6 week mark.
The best positions initially are on your back (for both men and women), or facing each other, with you lying on your strong side.
Be sure to avoid forcibly bending or twisting your knee.

Coping with Daily Activities

Some strategies to make the first few weeks at home a little easier...

Getting Dressed
- Sit down to get dressed.
- Put your operated leg into pants first, then your good leg.
- You may find long handled kitchen tongs help if you cannot bend your knee far enough for you to reach to your feet to slip on your pant legs.
- Reverse this procedure when removing pants or shorts.

Ironing
Preparation is key. Try to have all necessary ironing done prior to your hospital stay. In the first few weeks, have your support person iron if you really need it. If you don't have a support person to help you, try sitting on a high stool when ironing. If you sit - be careful to avoid a burn!

Carrying things around the house
Use a backpack to carry items around the house. If you must, you can hang a plastic bag over handle of your crutches.

Eating
To save you carrying your food, it is easier to eat at the bench on a stool rather than carry plates, cups and cutlery to the table.

Compression stockings
It is important to wear your compression stockings on both legs regularly and correctly to reduce your risk of developing deep vein thrombosis (DVT), otherwise known as blood clots, in your legs. You will be fitted in hospital for the correct size, based on your leg circumference and length. You must ensure that your stockings are correctly positioned around your toes, your heel, and that they do not cut in around the top of your leg. There must be no creases as these can also cut into your skin and leave a deep impression.

They can be a bit tricky to put on for the first few weeks. Ideally, your support person will be able to apply your stockings for you for the first 2 weeks or until you are confident. You have a few options when it comes to applying your compression stockings. It really comes down to personal preference as to which one you use:

- Wear rubber or latex kitchen gloves to increase your grip on the stockings. Bunch up the stocking as you would a normal sock. Slide this over your foot and position the toes correctly. Grasp the bunched stocking using the natural inward curve of the sole of your foot and pull it over your heel, positioning it correctly in the stocking. Lastly, grasp the stocking in the natural inward curve near your Achilles tendon and pull the remaining stocking length up and leg, ensuring no creases.
- For open-toe stockings - put your foot inside a plastic bag to reduce the friction as you slide the compression stocking over the top of the bag and up your leg. Once the stocking is in place, remove the bag via the open end at your toes.
- Ensure your legs are well moisturised to reduce friction of the stockings against the skin.
- You can use a special white "donning frame" if you have one, or if you simply cannot reach down far enough to your feet. These can be purchased from your local pharmacy if the options listed above are not successful.
- If all else fails, you may need to employ the service of a local home visit nursing organisation to apply the stockings after your shower each day. You should be independent with this after 2 - 3 weeks.

Hospital Packing List

The following items should be included in your hospital bag:
- Loose fitting shorts or pants that are easy to get on and off
- Comfortable, loose fitting shirts or blouses
- Underwear
- Warm cardigan or jumper - it can get very cold in the air conditioning
- Reading material
- Glasses
- Regular medication
- Slip on shoes (no lace-ups) with a non-slip sole
- Shoe horn
- Toiletries
    - toothbrush
    - toothpaste
    - hair brush or comb
    - moisturiser (very dry in the air conditioning)
    - deodorant or perfume
- Mobile phone and charger
- Medicare card
- Private Health card
- Purse with a small amount of cash only
- This book!

2

The Surgery

Explaining the Procedure

A total knee replacement is considered a major surgical procedure. Your surgery will usually take between 1 - 2 hours, roughly double this time for a bilateral procedure. Your surgical team will include your surgeon, an anaesthetist, junior doctors assisting and theater nurses.

The Prosthesis
Your new knee consists of 2 metal implants to replace the damaged ends of your femur (thigh bone) and tibia (shin bone); a plastic spacer that sits in between them to replace your removed knee meniscus (shock absorbing cartilage); as well as a plastic button which is used to resurface the underside of your patella (knee cap) if required.

Anaesthetic
Your anaesthetic will be tailored to your personal health circumstances. Generally, it will be a general anaesthetic, a spinal anaesthetic or a combination of the two. Your anaesthetist will select the most appropriate option based on your medical history and previous experiences with anaesthesia.

The Procedure
- Starting with an incision roughly 20cm long over the knee to expose your knee joint, your surgeon will move your soft tissue (ligaments, nerves and blood vessels) as well as your patella to one side.
- The damaged ends of your femur and tibia are removed and replaced with metal implants. The implants may be cemented in place, or may be designed to allow bone to grow into them to secure the metal to your bone.
- A plastic cushion sits in between the metal components to allow for smooth, frictionless movement of the joint.
- If the underside of the patella is damaged, it will be resurfaced with a plastic button.
- Your surgeon will use a computer to ensure optimal alignment of your new knee, and will double check your new joint is moving properly.

- Internal dissolvable stitches close up your joint, with staples or removable stitches closing the skin.

Recovery

You will wake in the recovery area with a bulky dressing covering your wound, as well as drainage tubes to help remove the swelling from the knee area. You may also have a urinary catheter in place for the first day or two. Compression stockings will have been applied in order to prevent blood clots forming in your legs.

Now the fun begins...

Medications

The medications you are prescribed by your surgeon play a vital role in your rehabilitation and long term recovery:
- They help you to complete your physiotherapy and exercise program properly. Thus improving your range and strength faster.
- They help you sleep better by reducing your pain overnight.
- They help you return to activity sooner by reducing your pain during the day.

However, many patients are under the misconception that they should wean off the pain relief as quickly as possible because:
- They are worried they will become addicted to the pain relief.
- They are concerned about the side effects of the pain relief.
- They "have a high pain threshold" and don't need the pain relief.
- They feel they are demonstrating their superior rehabilitation by telling their surgeon that they don't need pain relief.

Remember…you are undergoing a major surgical procedure. Without adequate pain relief it will hurt - a lot!

Prior to surgery, ensure you have told your surgeon about **ALL** the tablets/medication you take – even over the counter things like vitamins and supplements. These can impact on the drugs you are given in hospital. Make sure you also inform your surgeon of any allergies or bad reactions to any medication that you may have experienced in the past.

Main Medications
The main medications that you will be taking after surgery include:
- **Targin** (oxycodone & naloxone) - A slow release pain reliever that is taken morning and night. It contains naloxone which helps to block the side effects of oxycodone on your gut, such as constipation.

- **Endone** (oxycodone) - A fast release pain reliever that is taken for breakthrough pain throughout the day and night.
- **Paracetamol** (acetaminophen) - A pain reliever that works best when taken regularly.
- **Mobic** (meloxicam) - An anti-inflammatory medication taken daily with food to protect your stomach.
- **Xarelto** (rivaroxaban) - A blood thinner given to patients undergoing hip and knee replacements to help prevent blood clots (called DVT) in the leg.

Side Effects from Medications

Report the following side effects to your surgeon **immediately** as they may be **serious**:

- Vomiting, indigestion or abdominal pain
- Abnormal thinking or changes in mood, or feeling deep sadness
- Slow or noticeable heart beats
- Headache or confusion
- Drowsiness, feeling faint or fainting or dizziness especially when standing up
- Unusual weakness, loss of strength or trouble walking
- Urinary tract infections or changes in passing urine such as the volume passed, pain or feeling the need to urinate urgently.
- Breathlessness
- Chest pain
- Signs of allergic reaction such as:
    - rash, itching or hives on skin,
    - swelling of the face, lips, tongue, or other parts of the body,
    - shortness of breath, wheezing or trouble breathing
- Signs of liver problems such as yellowing of the skin and/or eyes (jaundice)
- Prolonged or excessive bleeding from gums, nose etc.
- Numbness in the arms and legs
- Heavy oozing of blood from a surgical wound
- Coughing up blood
- Blood in the urine or stool

- Heavy menstrual bleeding
- Signs of stroke such as:
    weakness in one part or side of your body,
    slurred speech,
    blurred vision or visual disturbances.

The following are possible side effects from your medications. Report them to your doctor if they worry you:
- *Nausea:* You can ask for an anti-emetic drug to stop you from feeling nauseated.
- *Constipation:* Eat a high fibre diet, try pear juice or prune juice, or speak with your local pharmacist.
- *Decreased appetite:* Often due to nausea or constipation. Eat small nutritious meals - little and often.
- *Feeling cloudy in the head*
- *Skin rash or itching*
- *Fatigue*
- *Dry mouth, hiccups, sore throat, thirst, trouble swallowing or changes in voice*
- *Anxiety or nervousness*
- *Trouble sleeping or abnormal dreams*
- *Excessive sweating, hot flushes*
- *Restlessness*
- *Muscle spasms, twitching or tremors*
- *Bruising*
- *Tinnitus (ringing in the ear)*

Weaning medications
Take your medications as instructed by your surgeon. Do not be in a hurry to wean yourself off your pain relievers. If you wean too early, you may suffer a setback to your recovery.
Generally the first pain reliever to stop is the Endone as it is for break through pain only. Most patients are in the process of weaning off their medications around 6 weeks. Some are weaning as early as week 4. It is important to speak with your surgeon at your 6 week review if you feel unable to wean off your pain medications.

Getting In & Out of Bed

It is easier to get in & out of bed on your strong side. Ensure your shoes and crutches or walking frame are within reach next to the bed.

Getting out of bed:
- Shift your body across the bed towards your strong side.
- Lower your strong leg over the side of the bed towards the floor.
- Use your arms to firstly prop up onto your elbows, and then push up towards sitting.
- As you are propping up on your arms, slide your operated leg over the side of the bed to rest your foot on the floor.
- You should now be sitting.

Getting into bed:
- Sit down on your strong side of the bed. For example, if you had a Right TKR, approach the RIGHT side of the bed **as you face it from the bottom of the bed**.
- Hook your strong foot underneath the ankle of your operated leg.
- Lean sideways onto the elbow of your strong side, as you swing your legs up onto the bed.

Roll onto your back and shift your body across to be in the middle of the bed.

Using Crutches

You will use your crutch/crutches in some capacity for up to 6 weeks. It is important that you correctly fit and use your crutches safely.
Incorrect fit can lead to neck and back pain. Poor crutch technique can lead to wrist pain or a fall and possibly damaging your new knee.

Fitting them to your height

The number of people who simply use the crutches as they find them is extraordinary. Crutches are adjustable so fit them to your height!

Axillary (or underarm crutches) are adjusted through the legs. Position the crutch 15 - 20cm outside your foot.
The correct fit is 2 - 3 fingers in between top of crutch and armpit. You can also adjust the height of the handle. Ideal handle height is when your elbow is bent to roughly 30 degrees.

Canadian crutches (or forearm/elbow crutches) can be adjusted through the legs for correct height, as well as at the top of the crutch for correct forearm length. To correctly fit for height, position the crutch 5 - 10cm outside your foot and 15cm in front. Your elbow should be bent between 15 - 30 degrees. Many new Canadian crutches have recommended height markers down the side. Adjust accordingly, but be willing to trial 1 level higher or lower until you find the height where you feel most comfortable. The cuff of the crutch is adjustable and should sit 3 - 4cm below the elbow.

Your shoulders should not be hunching upwards when you are using them. In this case, the crutches are *too high* and need to be adjusted to a lower height.

Equally, you should not be bending forwards or sideways when you are walking with them. In this instance, the crutches are *too low* and need to be adjusted higher.

Tie a ribbon/rubber band around one crutch

Many crutches have moulded grips for the left or right hands. You'll see an impressed L or R to indicate which crutch goes on which side. It is easier to tie a ribbon or a rubber band to one crutch, so you can quickly and easily spot which crutch is which.

Check stoppers

You should always check that the rubber stopper on the bottom of each crutch is not worn or covered in dirt/mud. They need to be nonslip as you are placing a fair amount of your body weight through them.

Walking technique

The crutches always go with your operated leg. In the instance of bilateral TKR - with the weaker of the two legs and this may change daily or even hourly.

The easiest way to start walking is to move both crutches and operated leg first, then step through with the good leg. Then repeat, repeat, repeat.
Don't rush! They can take a little while to get the hang of at first.

At first you may use a "step to" walking pattern. This means that after you step forward with your crutches and operated leg, you step your good leg forward to be in line with your operated leg.
As quickly as you can, progress yourself on to a "step through" walking pattern. This is where you swing your good leg past the operated leg as you move forward and is a more normal walking pattern.

Progress

Generally your progress will be 2 crutches - 1 crutch - 1 crutch outside only - none.

Initially you will leave hospital on 2 crutches. You will remain on 2 crutches inside and outside for 2-3 weeks.

At this time, as you get stronger and steadier, you may progress down to one crutch indoors. When you are using 1 crutch, it is important to use the crutch on your GOOD side.

Yes! When you progress on to one crutch, you will keep using the crutch on your non-operated side. The crutch still goes forward with the operated leg as you walk. This helps keep your walking smooth and balanced as you are shifting some of your weight off the operated leg towards the good side as you step through.

By 4 weeks you can usually stop using the crutch inside, and walk normally.

The progress outdoors is slower due to the distances you need to walk to get from place to place, the uneven surfaces you will encounter, as well as the general public. The crutches act as a visual reminder to the public to give you extra space.

Add 2 weeks on as a guide when progressing your crutch usage outdoors. For example, if you progressed from using both crutches to 1 crutch at 2 weeks, continue using 2 crutches outdoors until around 4 weeks.

Stairs

Stairs can create some anxiety for TKR patients. But they don't need to! When standing at the bottom of a flight of stairs - don't panic! Remember…

Good go to heaven…Bad go to Hell…

If you have a rail available, it can be easier to use the rail with one hand, and the crutch in the other. However, you will need to carry the spare crutch up under your arm to use once you get to the end of the stairs.

When going up stairs:
- Position your hand on the rail to be in line with the step you are traveling towards.
- Step up onto your good leg
- Then bring the crutches and operated leg up to the same step.

Repeat this for each step. In this way, you are using your stronger leg to control your balance and body weight.

Going down stairs is the reverse:
- If available, position your hand on the rail to be in line with the step you are travelling towards.
- Lead with your crutch(es) and operated leg at the same time. This allows you to control the descent with your stronger leg as it is the one lowering your body weight towards the next step.
- Once your crutches and operated leg are on the step, step down with your strong leg.

Troubleshooting

Sore wrists
You can get sore wrists with repetitive use of crutches, particularly in the first 2 weeks. Try to take more weight through your legs so there is less weight through your wrists. Limit the distance you walk and have regular breaks to move your hands/wrist/forearms and neck.

Sore neck
You can get a sore neck if the crutches have not be adjusted to the correct height. Read **Fitting them to your height** and adjust accordingly. Regularly move and stretch your neck, and apply warm packs for 20 minutes at a time whilst you are resting to help ease the aches.

Fear of stairs
You aren't usually discharged from hospital until you are confident on stairs, but sometimes fear of falling down stairs can be difficult to overcome. For some, standing at the top of a flight of stairs can be

overwhelming, and the natural reaction for these people is to freeze.
Read **Stairs** to ensure you know the correct technique.
Practice at only one step to begin with to build confidence with the basic technique.
Next, move onto 3 steps, with your partner or caregiver two steps in front of you. Don't look down to the bottom - instead, concentrate on one step at a time.
Now increase the number of steps you tackle. It won't take long until you are confident with a full flight of stairs. Practise, practise and practise again until stairs become second nature.

From Day 0 - Discharge

What to expect...

- **Mental Health:** You will be glad the surgery is over, but you are in the most difficult part of the recovery. You will be tired, sore and not too happy when your hospital physiotherapist arrives. You may be quite nervous for the first couple of walks, and the first time you try stairs.

- **Pain:** You will be on a lot of pain relief, but you have just had major surgery, so you will feel some pain on movement of your knee and when weight bearing. You may also feel pain around your thigh from where a surgical tourniquet has been applied. If you have access to Patient Controlled Anaesthesia (PCA) use it as you need. PCA is pain relief delivered when you press a button on a hand held device connected to pain medications delivered intravenously. Don't worry - you can't overdose when using a PCA as there is a lock out mechanism that uses a timer to prevent accidental overdose.

- **Swelling:** Your leg will appear quite swollen after the surgery from your mid-thigh down to your feet. You may have some bruising and notice that this bruising may migrate towards your feet and the back of your leg. This is due to gravity. You should use an ice pack to help reduce pain and swelling. The ice pack should be wrapped in a damp cloth and placed around your swollen knee. It should remain in place for 20 minutes. You may find the first 5 minutes of icing causes discomfort from the cold, but after that, your skin should be numbed and the discomfort will subside. There should be 2 hours between ice applications.

- **Stiffness:** Your knee will feel very stiff and difficult to move. This is due to your post-operative swelling. This is why it is so important to practise your exercises multiple times each day.

- **Mobility:** Depending on the time of your surgery, you will be walked either the same day, or early the following morning. You will have 2 physiotherapists and ward staff to help you. They will fit your new crutches and teach you how to use them correctly. Slowly but surely, they will increase the distance that you walk over the 4 - 7 days in hospital so that you will be able to cope at home.

- **Sleep:** You may not get much sleep at this point. Pain and discomfort in your leg may wake you. Being unable to sleep in your preferred position, as well as trying to sleep in an unusual bed with unusual sounds around you can also limit the amount of overnight sleep you achieve. Try to nap throughout the day where you can.

- **Physiotherapy:** If you had a morning procedure, you will meet your hospital physiotherapist during the afternoon. They will start your bed exercise program and teach you how to get in and out of bed, taking care of your drains and catheter bag and tubing. You will try going for a few steps with your crutches, but with loads of support from the physiotherapist and assistants. Over the coming days, they will work with you to improve the amount your knee bends and straightens, your safety on your crutches and your ability on stairs. Yes, we physiotherapists are bossy, but we truly want you to achieve your knee's full potential, so don't be too frustrated when you see us coming!

- **Exercises:** You will be instructed to perform regular breathing exercises, circulatory exercises and bed exercises designed to activate your quadriceps (thigh muscle) as it will be very weak after surgery. You will also need to practice bending your knee both in bed and when sitting. You may feel that your muscles will never move your leg again, but with regular practice and visualisation, your strength will slowly return.

- **Wound:** This will remain covered whilst in hospital with a bulky, waterproof dressing.

Risks and Complications
The main complications at this time are:
- *Blood clots:* You will be taking blood thinning medication and wearing your compression stockings to reduce this risk. It is important that you practice your circulatory exercises and move your knee little and often.

- *Infection:* Your wound is covered in a waterproof dressing to minimise this risk.

- *Falls:* Your risk of having a fall and damaging your new knee is highest whilst you are still getting used to your crutches. Make sure you call for assistance prior to getting out of bed during the first few days after surgery until your balance and confidence have improved.

Aims
- You will be discharged from hospital around day 4 – 5. This is usually once you can walk safely and have mastered stairs with your crutches.
- You will usually achieve 90 degrees of knee bend, but may not have full knee extension yet.
- You may not be able to straight leg raise or even really straighten your leg using your muscle strength at this time.

3

Your Exercise Program Explained

Why Your Exercise Program is Important...

You have invested a lot of time, pain and money into your new knee. It makes sense that you will want to get the very best out of it and have your knee reach its full potential. The best way to reach your knee's full potential is by following your exercise program.

Muscle Strength
Your leg, in particular, your quadriceps (thigh) muscle has been weakening for months prior to surgery due to the pain and stiffness you suffer with arthritis. You will have reduced the amount of exercise and general activity that you do to reduce your knee pain in order to "nurse" your knee through to surgery. The quadriceps muscles is very quick to lose its strength - after even 2 weeks of reduced use. Imagine the loss of strength after 6 - 12 months of low activity!

Immediately after surgery your leg is swollen, sore and your muscles are "pain inhibited". Pain inhibition is when your muscles are weaker, or don't seem to work well due to pain in and around that area. So, on top of your already weakened leg before surgery, you now have added weakness of your leg muscles due to the surgery itself.

Range of Motion
Performing your exercises regularly is vital to the complete recovery of full range of motion to your new knee. Full extension allows you to rest on your knee ligaments when you are standing, so not to rely on muscle strength to keep your knee stable. Full knee extension also helps you walk properly without a limp. Achieving excellent knee flexion range of motion is also important to a full recovery. Most knee replacements have the potential to achieve between 130 and 140 degrees of knee bend. As a guide, you need 110 degrees of bend to be able to clean between your toes and tie up your shoe laces. The more bend you have, the more activities you will be able to perform independently, easily and pain free.

Swelling
Regular movement of knee and more generally, your leg, provides a mechanical pump that reduces the swelling that travels down your leg with gravity. As the swelling reduces, so too, will your pain, and it will become easier to bend and straighten your knee.

Balance
Along with your muscle weakness, reduced activity and knee joint stiffness, the surgery itself will interfere with your ability to balance. Great balance is important as you get older to reduce your likelihood of falling. Your balance reduces every decade from the time you turn 40. A fall can be catastrophic to your new knee, so improving your balance is a very important part of your exercise program.

Endurance
Over the 12 months prior to the surgery, your reduced activity and pain will have led to a decrease in your endurance - your ability to walk as far you would like. Improving your endurance allows you to lead an active, healthy lifestyle for many years ahead.

Pain Management
The exercising of your knee, despite being painful at the time, is actually an excellent pain management strategy. As long as you follow an exercise plan that is "little and often", regular movement of your knee reduces swelling and stiffness and so reduces pain. However, overdoing your exercises will cause a spike in swelling, which stiffens your knee and increases your pain. So exercising moderately is the key!

Key Points Before You Start…

These are REALLY important to remember!!

- Pain relief is vital to successful rehabilitation. Time your pain relief to be taken 60 minutes prior to exercises to get the most benefit.

- Separate your bending and straightening exercises with at least 30 minutes in between. If you do them altogether, you will lose any gains made in each direction.

- Some days will be better than others, as long as the general direction is up. Listen to your body and don't get down if you aren't able to do "what the book says" today.

- Be flexible with the volume of exercise. If you wake up the next morning very sore and swollen, halve the volume of exercise and see how you are the next morning.

- Remember this is NOT a race. Moderation is the key. Don't compare yourself with others in the waiting room - as long as you achieve full recovery in the end.

If you would like a free 12 Week Exercise Planner to help keep track of your exercises, visit www.thetotalkneereplacement.com and enter your name and email address and you will receive a printable PDF in your in-box.

Overview of the Exercise Plan

The 12 week exercise plan included in this book contains a number of different exercises that are introduced at key points throughout your 12 week recovery period. It is important to understand how these different types of exercise contribute to your recovery.

1. Stretching

Stretching the muscles of your lower leg helps to reduce muscle tightness and improve the range of motion of your new knee. The key areas to stretch are:
- Calf
- Quadriceps
- Hamstrings
- Lower back and Buttocks

Stretches should be held for 30 seconds to allow the muscle enough time to relax and lengthen. It is better to perform one long stretch properly, than it is to perform 5 x shorter stretches. You should feel a stretch sensation, rather than pain. If it is painful, stop. Reposition so that you feel the stretch sensation instead.

2. Strengthening

Strengthening your muscles after knee surgery is vital to your recovery. The key areas you need to strengthen are:
- Quadriceps
- Calf
- Gluteals
- Hamstrings
- Hip Abductors

Ensure you strengthen both legs as you will have de-conditioned on both sides due to reduced activity. You can also perform general body strengthening exercises for your back, upper body and arms.

If you are returning to work or an approved sport, you can also include specific exercises for these tasks later into your recovery.

3. Walking

You will start a progressive walking program from Day 1. Initially you will walk with 2 crutches inside on flat, firm surfaces. Slowly you will increase your time and distance.
Once you are confident and safe, you will progress to using only 1 crutch - in the hand of your strong (non-operated) side.

Even with crutches, it is important that you try to walk reasonably quickly. It is safer than walking slowly as all your energy is moving forwards rather than sideways. You do not have time to limp!

You will begin walking short distances outside on flat ground. Slowly increase your time by adding on an extra driveway or light pole each walk. However, be sure to not increase your distance too quickly as you can suffer a setback, with increased swelling, resulting in stiffness and pain.

Always use an extra level of safety outside. For example, if you are using 1 crutch indoors, still use 2 crutches outside to protect against uneven ground, longer distances between rest stops and the general public who may bump into you if they are not paying attention.

Options to extend your walking program include introducing short inclines or trying the same distance but at a faster speed.

Once you no longer require crutches, make sure to swing your arms as they help keep you balanced when you are walking.

4. Balance

Your balance actually begins to decline from age 40. Most people don't notice their poor balance until it is tested or until they fall. Your balance is the combination of information from your vision, your inner ear and nerve endings (proprioceptors) in your feet that tell your brain your body's position in space. It is also influenced by a variety of factors, such as your medications, the surrounding environment and your confidence.

A fall could seriously damage your new knee, so balance exercises are an important component of your exercise program.

Some balance exercises include:
- Stand on 1 leg with your eyes open. Aim for 30 seconds on each leg. Most people over 80 years can only manage 3 seconds.
- Now do it with your eyes closed. This replicates night time. Do this near a bench or solid chair for safety, as it is more challenging when you can't rely on your vision for feedback.
- Now stand on 1 leg on an uneven surface such as grass or sand.
- Simply walking backwards without holding on is a great balance exercise. Have someone watching you until you are confident that you are safe.
- Try walking heel-toe forwards along a line.
- Walk heel-toe backwards along the line.

5. Exercise Bike

An exercise bike can be a great way to provide repetitive, non-weight bearing bending of your knee. Initially you should ensure the exercise bike has the highest possible seat position with no resistance to the pedals. You could also try a set of pedals that sits on the ground whilst you remain seated in your chair.

Progress your exercise by increasing the time on the bike first. As you cope with increased time, try lowering the seat height, one notch at a time. This will increase the knee bend at the top of the pedal.

Lastly, try to slowly and gradually increase the resistance to the pedals. This will help to improve your leg strength.

6. Hydrotherapy

Hydrotherapy is a great exercise option for total knee replacement rehabilitation patients once their wound is completely healed.

Look for an appropriate pool which is:
- Heated
- Has a ramp with a rail to hold onto for easy entrance and exit
- Is at least as deep as your chest.

It is advisable to check with your local pool regarding the best times to go, as you don't want to be exercising alongside toddler swimming lessons!

Hydrotherapy sessions should initially be 20 minutes long only. It won't seem like much, but it is very easy to overdo things, and afterward, you will feel exhausted. You can do all your land based exercises in the water.

You can increase the difficulty by moving faster through the water. This creates extra turbulence and improves your strength. Equally, you can make exercises easier by slowing down the movement and reducing the turbulence around you. The addition of things such as paddles, weights, stretchy bands, pool noodles or buoyancy vests increases the effort you need to complete the program of exercises.

A basic hydrotherapy program will include:
- Warm up - Walking forwards, backwards and sideways.
- Strengthening - Calf raises, butt kicks, squats, lunges, marching, swing leg out to the side.
- Balance - Stand on one leg with eyes open and closed. Extend this by creating turbulence with your arms. You can also walk heel-toe forwards and backwards.

You can progress, as appropriate, with the use of the equipment listed above. Remember, the bigger the surface area of the paddle, the greater the resistance and the more challenging the exercise.

4

Exercises and Expectations from Discharge to 12 weeks & beyond

From Discharge - Week 2

What to expect...

The first 2 weeks are the most difficult. **Remember - you have just had Major Surgery!**

- **Mental Health:** You will be quite happy to be through the surgery and hospitalisation and back home in your own bed! You will look forward to seeing your physiotherapist to double check how you are going with your exercises. You will also look forward to seeing your Surgeon on Day 14 to remove the staples and have a good look at the wound site. You may be a bit concerned at how your knee seems to have stiffened a bit since your discharge. As always, speak with your Surgeon and Physiotherapist about any concerns.

- **Pain:** You will be sore from the surgery, so it is vital that you take your pain medications as directed to ensure your successful rehabilitation following surgery. You will be on some strong pain relief medication for the next few weeks. People react differently to these medications - you may feel nauseated or feel cloudy in your head from the pain medication. Continue taking the medications, but speak with your Surgeon if this concerns you.

- **Swelling:** Your knee will be swollen. Swelling increases both the pain and stiffness of your knee. It is important that you move your knee little and often, and ice and elevate your leg in between to help reduce the swelling. You may find ice is helpful in reducing pain and swelling around the knee. Remember – 20 minutes ON and at least 2 hours OFF. Your knee area may feel warm for a few months. This is normal. You will be expected to wear compression stockings on both legs for 6 weeks after your surgery. These will help to limit the amount of swelling in your lower legs and reduces your risk of developing a blood clot.
- **Stiffness:** You may actually lose some range of motion in the first 2 weeks after discharge from hospital. This happens to

most patients. Now that you are home, even with a fantastic Support Network, you will slowly be doing more and more. This will increase your swelling and knee pain and lead to some stiffening up of your knee. Performing your exercises as directed will help ease the stiffness. Improving knee extension is the primary aim for the first few weeks.

- **Mobility:** You will continue to use 2 crutches, and will still be getting used to using them. They may make your wrists sore, so try not to lean on them so heavily. Your knee is safe to bear your weight. You will remain mostly inside during this time. A good tip is to tie a ribbon or rubber band around one crutch, so you can easily work out which side is which. Do not overdo your walking at this stage! It will come back slowly but surely. Too much walking will cause you pain, swelling and actually stiffen your knee.

- **Sleep:** You will feel very tired. This will last for 4 – 5 weeks. This is normal with any major surgery. You will generally be sleeping on your back at this time. If your leg is especially swollen, you can have your knee positioned on a pillow for support and mild elevation. If you aren't used to sleeping on your back, you may not sleep well. Equally, your knee pain may wake you up through the night. You can try gently bending it back and forth 10 times to reduce any pain and stiffness, or take extra pain relief through the night and this may aid in your return to sleep. Getting a good night sleep really helps you cope with your knee pain much better during the day, so do what you can to get enough rest overnight.

- **Physiotherapy:** Make an appointment to see your Physiotherapist around day 7-10 for your first consultation after discharge from hospital. They will check your understanding of your exercises, check you are safely using your crutches and answer any questions you may have at this time. They will monitor your wound, your knee's range of movement and check your lower leg for any sign of blood clots. You should arrange to see them either weekly or twice per week depending on how much motivation you need with your recovery. Generally patients either perform their exercises too little or too often. Please follow your physiotherapist's advice and perform them as directed. This provides the best outcome for your knee.

- **Exercises:** You should perform the basic exercises 3 x day. You may find performing a Straight Leg Raise difficult at this time. Don't be disheartened - your Quads strength will return with regular practice. Separate your exercises into the ones that "Bend" your knee and those that "Straighten" your knee. Do the Bending ones in a group. Then, 30 – 45 minutes later, do the Straightening exercises. You'll get better, longer lasting results. Time your exercises to start one hour after you have taken your fast acting pain relievers to allow you to exercise relatively pain-free.

- **Wound:** You will have any Staples out at 2 weeks and your Surgeon or Practice Nurse will check your wound. They will replace your waterproof dressing at this time. Make sure that if you need to replace your own wound dressing, to bend your knee as much as possible before applying the waterproof dressing. Please don't touch your wound at this stage until it is fully closed.

Aims for Week 2

- **Exercises** - Perform 3 x day. Be able to lift your leg up off the bed by Day 14.
- **Knee flexion** - Maintain 90 degrees of knee bend through to Day 14.
- **Knee extension** - Be within 10 degrees of full extension.
- **Mobility** - Safely use 2 crutches indoors and up & down stairs as needed. Minimal outside walking.

Risks & Complications

The main complications at this time are:

- Blood clots – You will be taking blood thinning medication and wearing your compression stockings to reduce this risk. It is important that you move about little and often.

- Infection – Your wound is covered in a waterproof dressing through this time to minimise this risk. Do not touch your wound. If the dressing comes off, call your doctor's surgery to arrange a new one. When applying a new dressing, bend your knee as much as you can before putting on the new dressing.

- Falls - Your risk of having a fall and damaging your new knee is highest whilst you are getting used to your crutches. Make sure you have clear passageways through your home, and be sure to slow down when using your crutches during this time.

Exercise Program - The First Week

Circulatory exercises

The following exercises are performed to help improve the circulation in your legs after surgery in order to prevent the formation of a deep vein thrombosis (blood clot).

- **Buttock squeezes -**
Position: Lay on the bed face up. Legs are out straight.
Action: Tighten your buttock muscles for 3 seconds and then relax.
Repeat: 10 times.
Frequency: Hourly.

- **Thigh squeezes -**
Position: Lay on the bed face up. Legs are out straight.
Action: Tighten your thigh muscles (quadriceps) and then relax.
Repeat: 10 times.
Frequency: Hourly.

- **Ankle pumps -**
Position: On the bed, face up; or sitting on a chair.
Action: Move your foot up and down at the ankle joint. Pull your toes and foot up and then point your toes and foot down.
Repeat: 10 times.
Frequency: Hourly.

Breathing exercises

The following exercises are designed to ensure your lungs remain fully inflatable and to prevent the development of a chest infection.

1. Deep breathing -
Position: On the bed, face up; or sitting in a chair.
Action: Rest your hands on the very bottom of your ribcage. Take a slow, long, deep breath in through your nose. Breathe in so that the lowest parts of your ribcage are expanding out into your hands. Ensure your shoulders don't rise up towards your ears - that is shallow breathing and we want to avoid that.
Repeat: 5 breaths
Frequency: Hourly.

2. Tri-flow - A device provided by your hospital that may consist of coloured balls, or a slider to encourage long, deep breaths.
Position: Seated in a chair.
Action: Sit with good posture. Breathe all the way out. Position the mouthpiece securely in your mouth with your lips forming a good seal. Take a long deep breath in, filling the bottom of your lungs with air. Hold momentarily, then breathe out.
Repeat: 5 breaths.
Frequency: Hourly.

Bed exercises

The bed exercises are designed to improve the range of movement and strength of your knee. You should perform all the exercises that involve bending your knee separately to those that straighten your knee. Leave a 30 minute gap in between the bending and straightening exercises. Try to perform these 3 x day if you can.

Straightening
1. Thigh squeeze

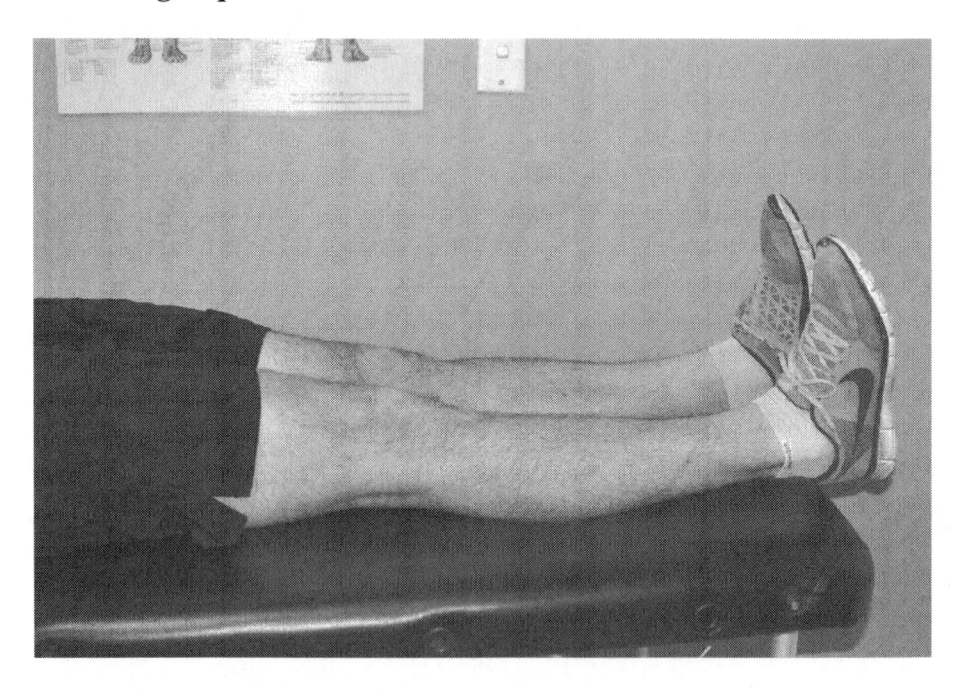

Position: Lay on the bed face up. Legs are out straight.
Action: Tighten your thigh muscles (quadriceps) and then relax.
Repeat: 10 times.
Frequency: 3 x day.
Note: Your thigh muscle may feel very soft, as if it is not working, at this early stage due to pain inhibition. Persist with this exercise regardless.

2. Straight leg raise

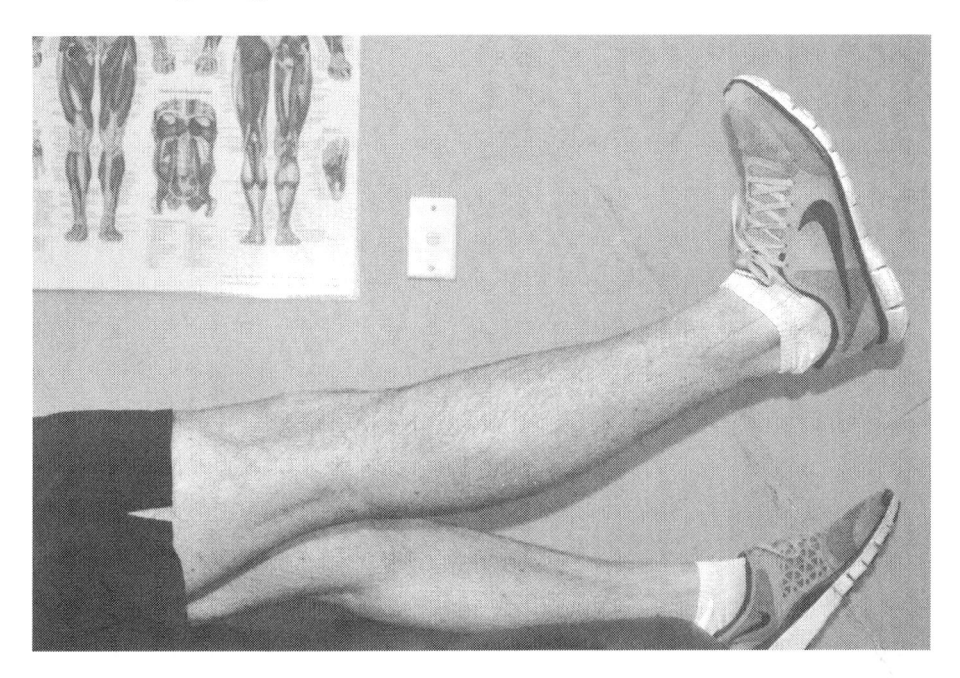

Position: Lay on the bed face up. Legs are out straight.
Action: Tighten your thigh muscles (quadriceps). Visualise your kneecap (patella) moving towards your hip, and the heel of your foot pressing out away from you. Toes should be pulled back towards you. Lift your straight leg up off the bed about 30cm, then slowly lower it back to the bed and relax.
Repeat: 10 times.
Frequency: 3 x day.
Note: Some patients are unable to actually lift their leg off the bed until around Day 10 - 14. So if you cannot perform this exercise well in Week 1 - don't worry! Persist and you will get there.

3. Inner range quads

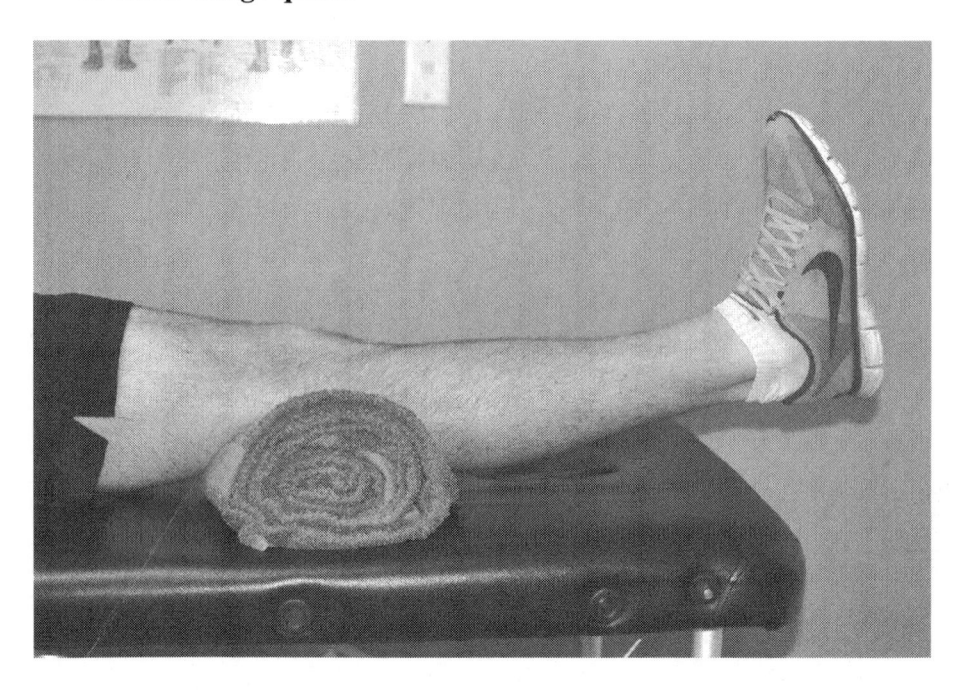

Position: Lay on the bed face up. Position a rolled up towel under your knee.

Action: Tighten your thigh muscles (quadriceps). Visualise your kneecap (patella) moving towards your hip, and the heel of your foot pressing out away from you. Toes should be pulled back towards you. Keep the underside of your knee on the rolled towel. Lift your lower leg up off the bed until your knee is straight, then slowly lower it back to the bed and relax.

Repeat: 10 times

Frequency: 3 x day.

Note: You may not be able to get your knee perfectly straight for some time. Don't worry! Just keep practicing.

4. Passive knee extension over roll

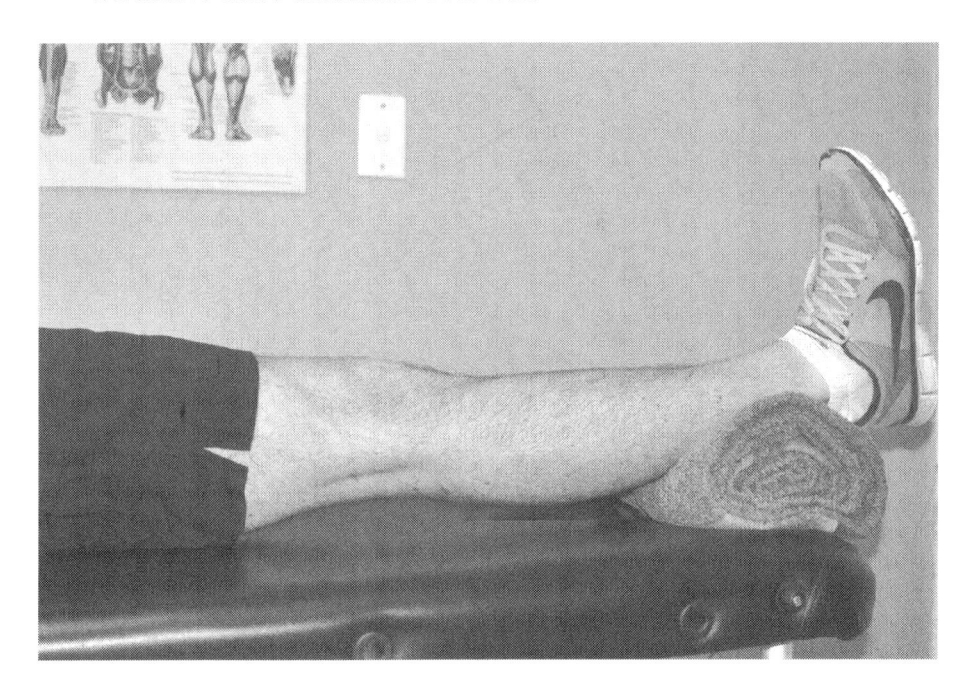

Position: Lay on the bed face up. Position the rolled towel under your ankle. Keep your toes pointing to the ceiling - don't allow your leg to roll in or out.
Action: Relax your leg and allow gravity to help straighten your knee. Hold for 2 minutes if able.
Repeat: Once per session.
Frequency: 3 x day.
Note: Some patients are directed to perform this for 5 minutes, but find holding this position for that length of time very painful. Just do what you can cope with. You can build up the time later as you tolerate it better.

Bending
5. Heel slide

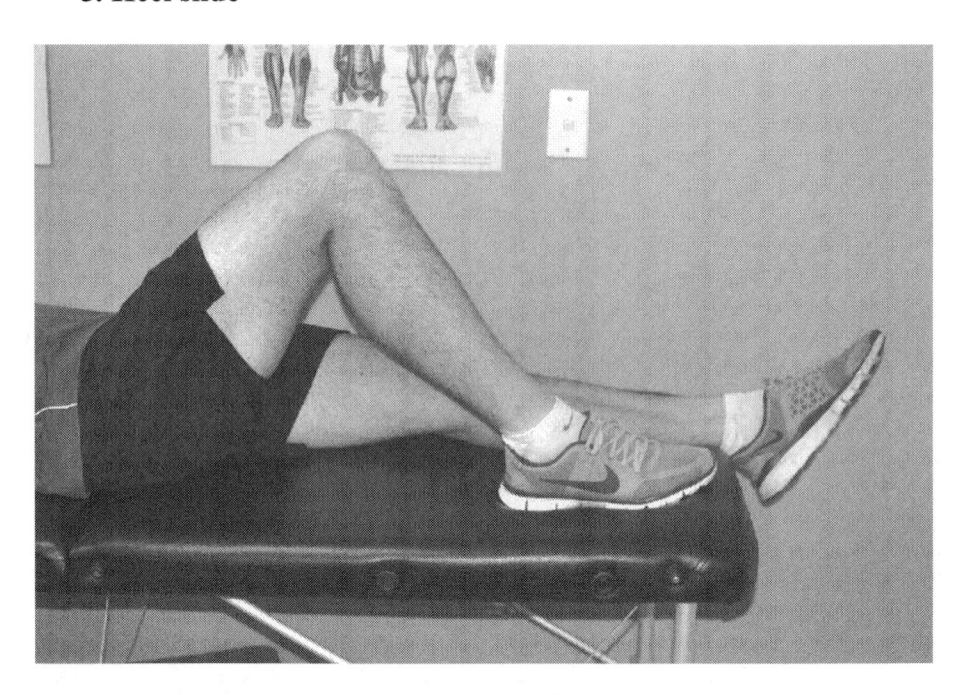

Position: Lay on the bed face up. Legs are out straight.
Action: Slide your heel towards your bottom as far as you can. Hold momentarily, then slowly straighten out your leg and relax.
Repeat: 10 times.
Frequency: 3 x day.
Note: You may find it easier with a large plastic bag under your foot to reduce the friction of the bed coverings.

Seated Exercises

Straightening
1. Seated knee extension

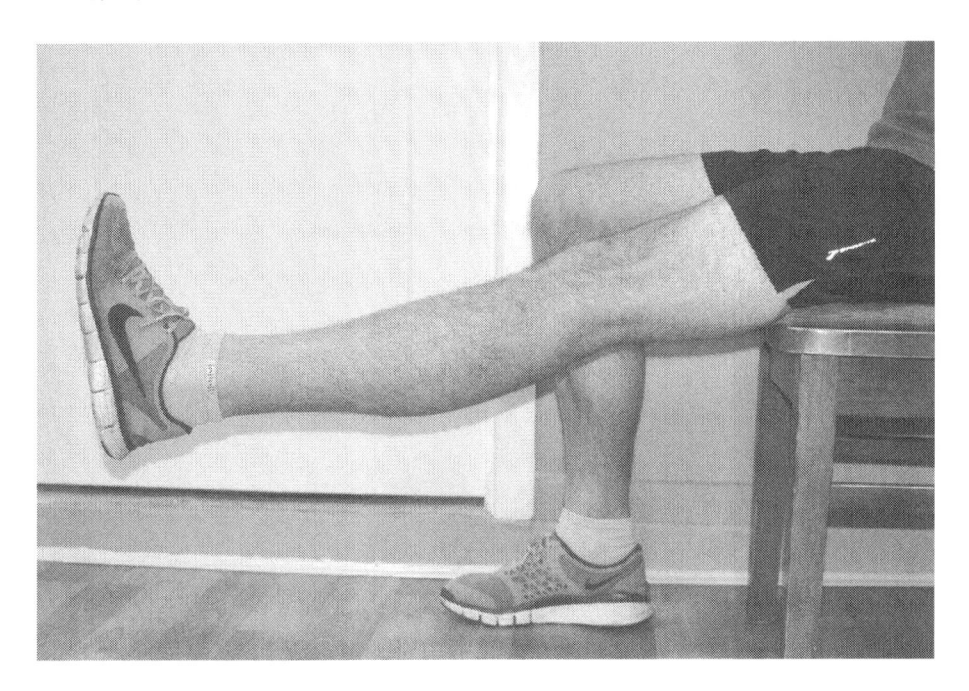

Position: Seated on a high, firm chair.
Action: Slowly straighten your knee until it is locked straight (or as straight as you can get it). Hold momentarily and then lower slowly.
Repeat: 10 times.
Frequency: 3 x day.
Note: You may feel a stretch sensation at the back of your knee or calf muscle.

Bending
2. Seated knee bend

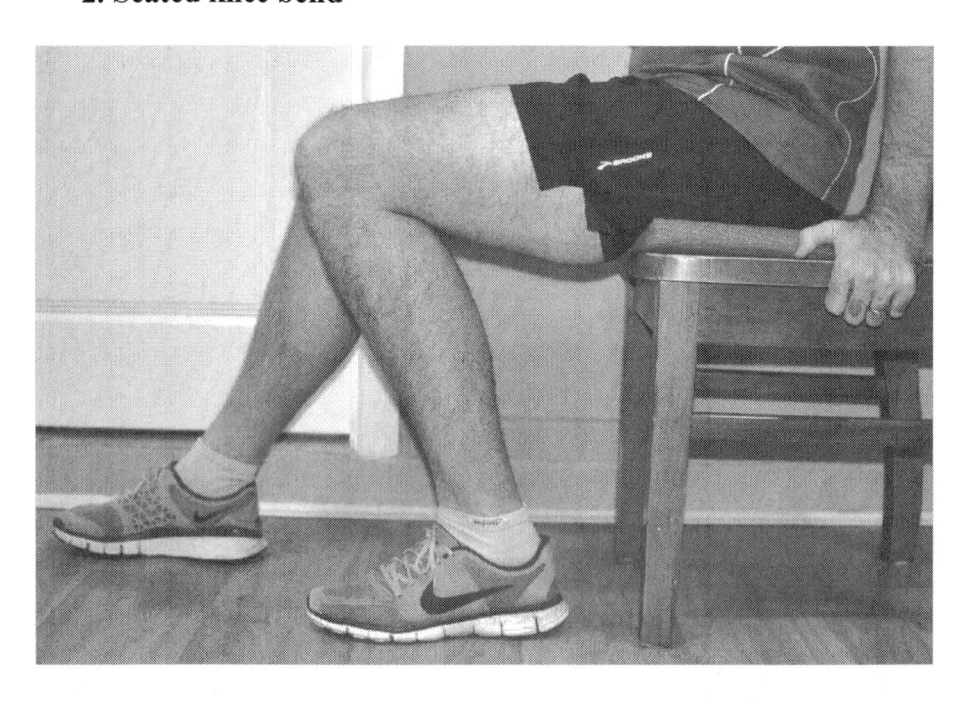

Position: Seated on a high, firm chair.
Action: Slide your foot backwards under the chair. Hold momentarily and then slide your foot back to its original position. You can also try using your good leg to help, by crossing it over your operated leg's ankle and pulling your operated foot backwards.
Repeat: 10 times.
Frequency: 3 x day.
Note: During the first week you will only be able to achieve roughly 90 degrees due to pain, swelling, staples and wound dressings. You may use a large plastic bag under your foot to reduce friction and improve your sliding action.

Walking

Walk using both crutches around the inside of your home only this week. Do this little and often, with a good rest in between. Refer to the page Using Crutches.

Stairs

Practice going up and down stairs if you have them at home, only when you have someone with you this week. Refer to the page Using Crutches for the safest method.

Exercise Program - The Second Week

Circulatory exercises - Continue performing these exercises hourly.
- Buttock squeezes
- Thigh squeezes
- Ankle pumps

Breathing exercises - Continue to perform these exercises hourly.
- Deep breathing
- Tri-flow

Bed exercises - Continue to perform these 3 x day. You should see the improvement in your straight leg raise this week. Continue to separate your exercises into those that bend and those that straighten.
- Thigh squeezes
- Inner range quads
- Straight leg raise
- Passive knee extension over roll
- Heel slides

Seated Exercises - Continue to perform these 3 x day.
- Seated knee extension
- Seated knee bend

Walking - Continue to walk indoors little and often. You will be more confident with your crutches.

Stairs - You should be a little more confident on stairs this week. Continue to practise if you have them at home.

Bench exercises
Straightening
1. Calf raises

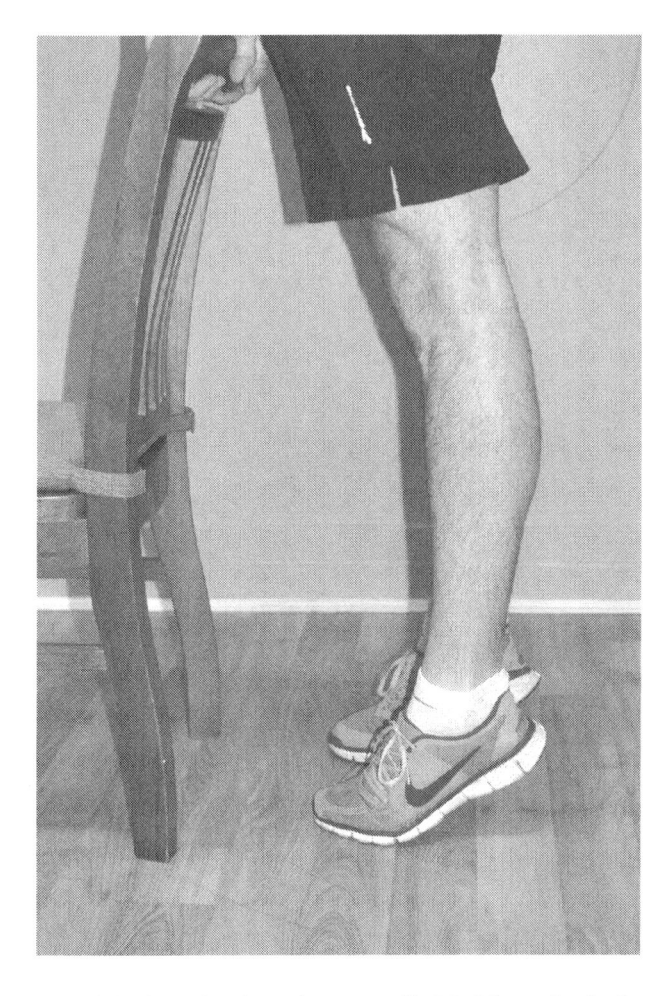

Position: Stand facing the bench or a rail. Hold on for balance.
Action: Rise up onto your toes so that your heels are up off the ground. Lower slowly, then rock back onto your heels, lifting your toes up off the ground.
Repeat: 10 times.
Frequency: 3 x day.
Note: Everyone enjoys this exercise!

2. Swing leg out to the side

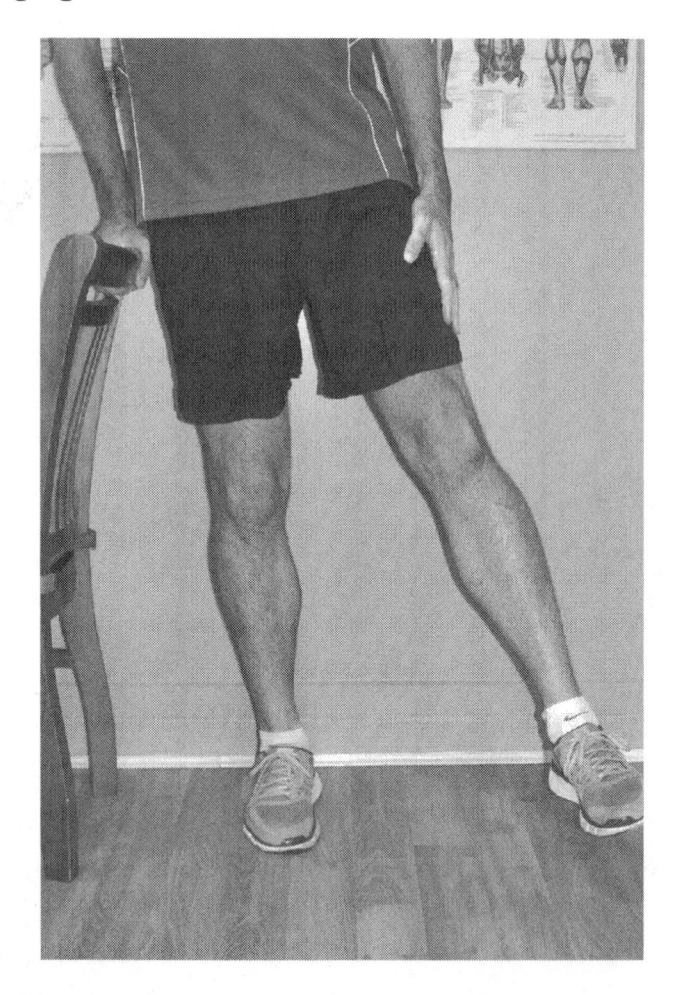

Position: Stand facing the bench or a rail. Hold on for balance and support.
Action: Standing tall, in good posture, swing your leg out to the side, away from your body.
Repeat: 10 times in a row on one leg, then 10 times on the other leg.
Frequency: 3 x day.
Note: Ensure your toes remain pointing forward so that your leg doesn't rotate outward during the movement.

Bending
1. March on spot

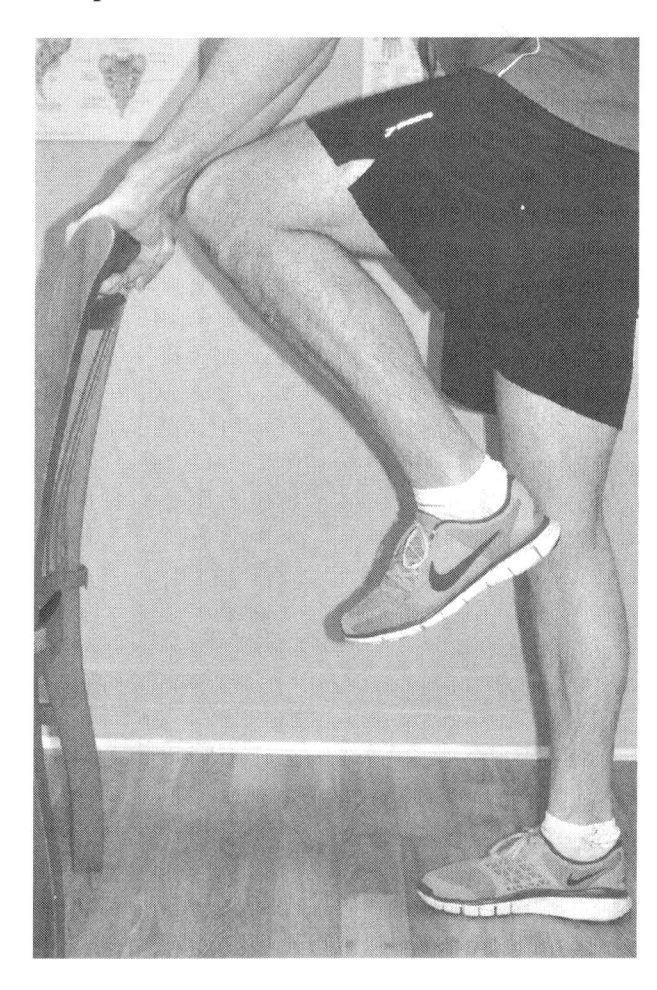

Position: Stand facing the bench or a rail. Hold on for balance and support.
Action: March on the spot, lifting your knees up towards hip height.
Repeat: 10 times each leg (20 steps in total)
Frequency: 3 x day
Note: If it is too painful to stand on your operated leg when raising your good knee, just lift your operated leg for now.

2. Kick butt

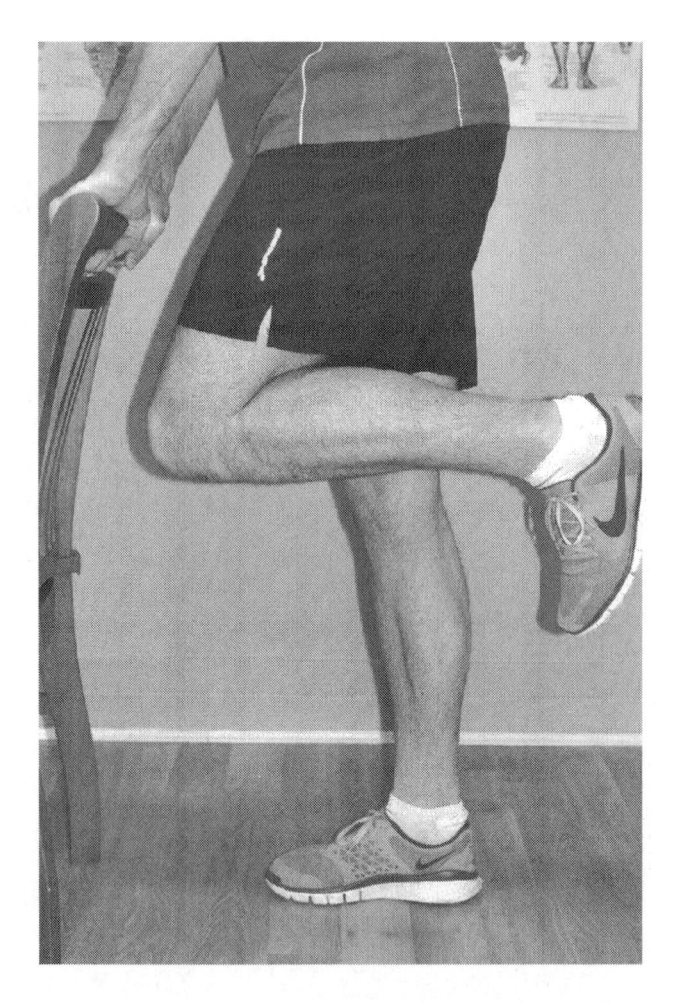

Position: Stand facing the bench or a rail. Hold on for support.
Action: Allow your knee to move forward slightly. Pull your toes up toward you. Flick your heel up towards your buttocks, then lower back to the ground.
Repeat: 10 times.
Frequency: 3 x day.
Note: Most people find this the most challenging exercise, so don't be concerned if you can't raise your foot very far this week.

3. Shallow squat

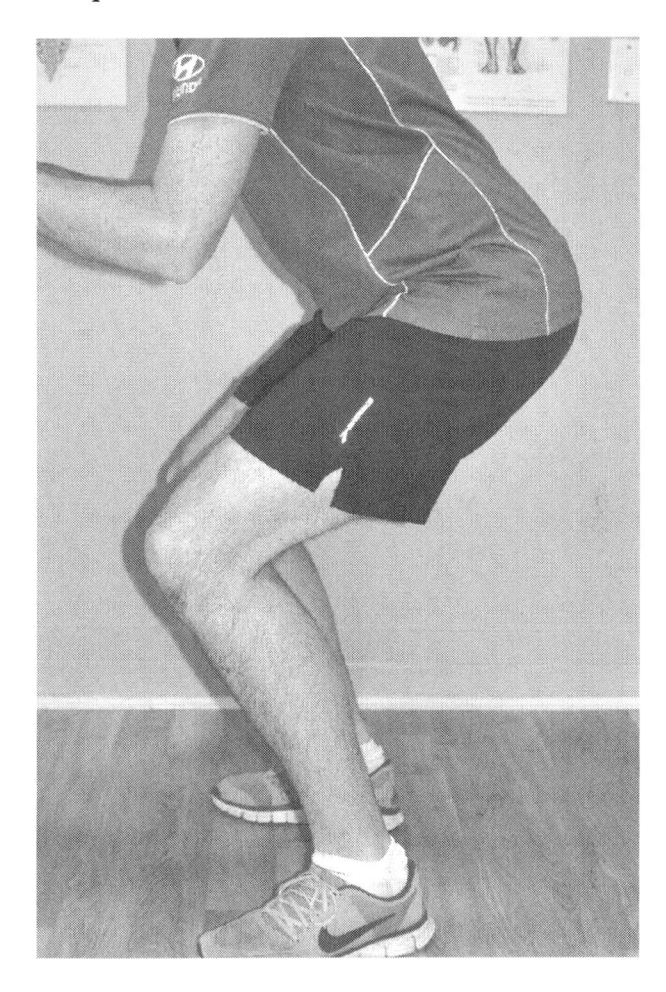

Position: Stand facing the bench or a rail. Hold on for support. Feet are positioned under each hip.

Action: Pretend that you are sitting down. Lean forward whilst sticking your buttocks backward. Allow your knees to bend towards a quarter to half squat. Then stand up straight.

Repeat: 10 times (or as able).

Frequency: 3 x day.

Note: If shallow squats are too painful or you feel that they are too much for now, replace this exercise with sit to stand.

4. Sit to Stand

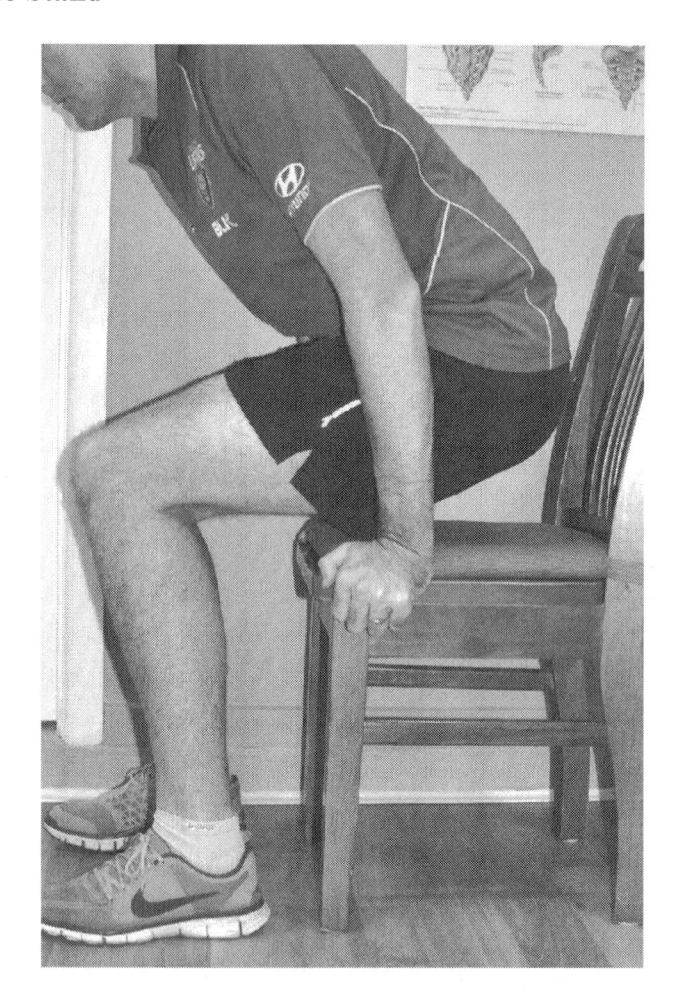

Position: Stand in front of a high, firm chair.
Action: Lean forward through your hips, sticking your bottom backwards as you sit down. Then stand up again.
Repeat: 10 times (or as able).
Frequency: 3 x day.
Note: You should find this exercise more suitable if the squat is too difficult for now. You may use the arm rests if you need.

Weeks 2 – 4

What to expect...

- **Mental Health:** Weeks 2 - 4 are the most difficult. You may feel flat, frustrated or even teary towards the end of the 4th week due to a combination of fatigue, cabin fever and frustration at perceived lack of progress. This can be quite concerning for you or your family, but is very common. Don't be too hard on yourself (or your Support Network)! Make sure you get out of the house and grab a coffee. Have your Support Network park the car close to the café and enjoy being outside in the fresh air!

- **Pain:** You will still be sore, but the level of pain will slowly be decreasing. You may find that you are having good days and bad days. Usually, on good days, you tend to overdo things and so cause extra pain and swelling the following day. It is important that you continue to take your pain medications as directed to ensure your successful rehabilitation following surgery. You may wish to <u>begin</u> phasing out your pain medications slowly towards the end of this fortnight. Please note: stopping pain medication too soon can setback your rehabilitation by a week or more. Generally the short acting pain reliever will be the first to be reduced. However, you may still need to take these an hour prior to your physiotherapy sessions. You may also need to take one every now and then after you have overdone things. This is not a setback. It is simply a reminder to do things in moderation.

- **Swelling:** Your knee swelling will slowly reduce. You will notice that your knee swells up during the day whilst you are up and about, but reduces in size overnight as you sleep. Try to get your household tasks done in the morning, so that you can ice and elevate your legs through the afternoon. You will be getting frustrated with your compression stockings - please continue to wear them as directed!

- **Stiffness:** Your knee stiffness will fluctuate hour to hour and day to day. However, overall, there will be an improvement to both your knee bending and straightening. Once you are able to fully extend your knee, your primary focus turns to improving your knee bend. You can now start using the skateboard - see **Exercises** below. It is such an easy way to improve your knee bend without as much pain.

- **Mobility:** You will progress down to using just one crutch indoors - the crutch on your **strong** side. You may even start to walk a few steps without support, especially in the kitchen and areas where you have furniture you can lean on for support. You will still need to use 2 crutches outdoors for this period. Mobilising outdoors is more risky due to the uneven surfaces, the greater distances between seats/rest stops, and the chance that you may be accidentally knocked over by a member of the general public. You may slowly increase the distance you walk this fortnight. Start with going for a walk for 5 - 10 minutes. Do not rush to improve your walking distance yet! Too much walking at this stage will still cause you pain, swelling and knee stiffness.

- **Sleep:** You will still feel very tired and this can really affect your mood. You may still be struggling to achieve a good night's sleep. This is normal and should improve by Week 4. If you are particularly distressed due to lack of sleep, please speak with your Family Doctor who may be able to prescribe a sleeping tablet if all other strategies have been unsuccessful.

- **Physiotherapy:** You will continue to see your Physiotherapist weekly. They will continue to monitor your knee's range of movement; wound site; and check for any blood clots. They will check your exercise technique, and progress your exercise program as you improve. Your Physiotherapist will advise when you can progress to one crutch and commence a graduated walking program.

- o **Exercises:** Time to grab your skateboard! Sit on a chair in your kitchen (or other hard surfaced area). Place the skateboard on the ground and put the foot of your operated leg on it. Move the skateboard back and forth to gently and easily increase your knee bend. Do this for 2 – 3 minutes at a time. You will progress onto weight bearing exercises performed at your kitchen bench. You will continue to perform your exercises 3 x day. Continue to separate your exercises into the bending and straightening exercises.

- o **Wound:** Your wound will no longer need the waterproof dressing from roughly week 3. If there is any localised area of skin separation along the scar line, you may use a steri-strip to hold the sides of the wound together. Until the wound is fully closed, please avoid touching the scabs or entering a swimming pool.

Aims for Week 4

- o **Exercises** - Perform 3 x day. You will progress onto weight bearing exercises.
- o **Knee flexion** - Achieve 90 - 100 degrees of bend by Week 4.
- o **Knee extension** - Be within 5 degrees of full extension. Straight leg raise is much easier.
- o **Mobility** - You will progress down to one crutch indoors by the end of 4 weeks. You are slowing increasing the outside distance you can walk. You will still need 2 crutches outside at this time.

Risks & Complications

The main complications at this time are:
- o Blood clots – Please continue to wear your compression stockings and monitor your lower leg for signs of a blood clot.

- o Infection – Your wound cover is off from the middle of this fortnight. Please still avoid touching the wound site. Please continue to monitor for signs of infection.

- Stiffness - Your knee will stiffen up if you overdo your walking and exercises. This is not a race! Perform your rehabilitation at a moderate pace and you will enjoy a full recovery.

Exercise Program - Week 3

Circulatory exercises - You can reduce these exercises to 3 x day provided your swelling is reducing.
- Buttock squeezes
- Thigh squeezes
- Ankle pumps

Breathing exercises - Reduce these exercises to 3 x day provided you do not have any chest conditions or infections.
- Deep breathing
- Tri-flow

Bed exercises - Continue to perform these 3 x day.
- Thigh squeezes
- Inner range quads
- Straight leg raise
- Passive knee extension over roll
- Heel slides

Seated Exercises - Continue to perform these 3 x day.
- Seated knee extension
- Sit to stand
- Seated knee bend - You can now introduce a skateboard under your foot instead of the plastic bag to improve your bend.

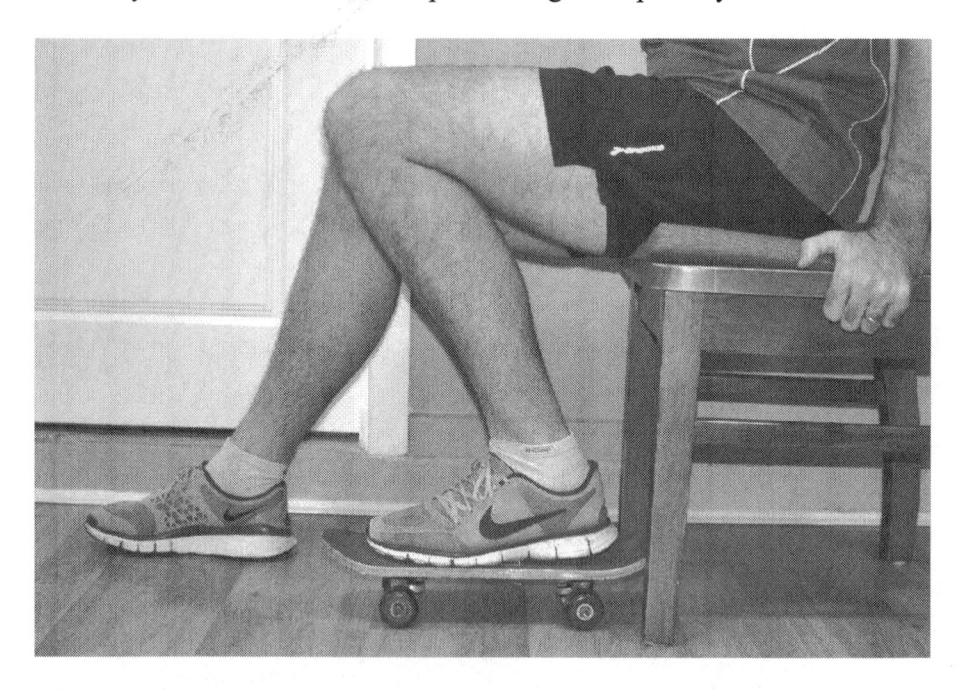

Walking - Continue to walk indoors little and often. This week try going out for a coffee or other very short outing to gradually begin walking outdoors.

Stairs - Continue to practice these daily if you have them at home.

Bench exercises - Continue to perform these 3 x day.
- Calf raises
- Swing leg out to the side
- March on spot
- Kick butt
- Shallow squat

Stretches
- **Calf stretch**

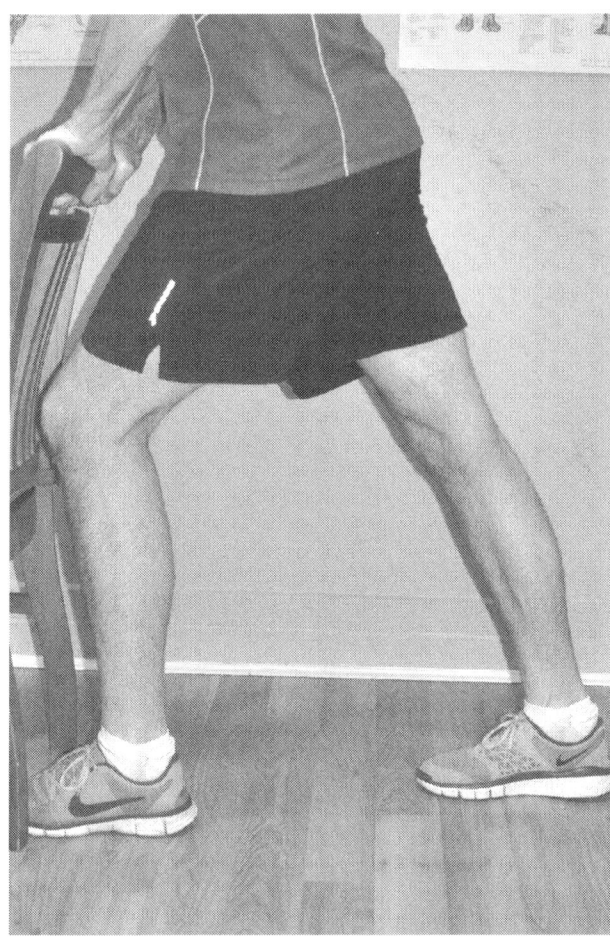

Position: Stand at a bench. Move one foot forward and keep the other foot in place. Both feet are facing forwards.

Action: Lean forwards onto your front foot, allowing the front knee to bend. The heel of the back foot remains flat on the ground. The knee of the back leg remains straight. Feel the stretch behind the knee and down the back of lower leg (calf muscle).

Repeat: Hold the stretch for 30 seconds. Swap legs and perform on the other side.

Frequency: 3 x day.

Note: This stretches the back leg. Do this stretch on both legs.

Exercise Program - Week 4

Circulatory exercises - You can reduce these exercises to 3 x day provided your swelling is reducing.
- Buttock squeezes
- Thigh squeezes
- Ankle pumps

Bed exercises - Continue to perform these 3 x day.
- Thigh squeezes
- Inner range quads
- Straight leg raise
- Passive knee extension over roll
- Heel slides

Seated Exercises - Continue to perform these 3 x day.
- Seated knee extension
- Seated knee bend with skateboard.
- Sit to stand

Walking - Begin walking outdoors for distance. Start with a daily 10 minute walk and gradually increase the time as able. As a guide, try to increase your walk time by 5 minutes per week. You will need 1 - 2 crutches for your outdoors walk. Aim to walk quickly, as this will reduce any limp and normalise your gait pattern.

Stairs - Continue to practice these daily if you have them at home. You may be able to progress to one foot per step this week.

Bench exercises - Continue to perform these 3 x day.
- Calf raises
- Swing leg out to the side
- March on spot
- Kick butt
- Shallow squat

Stretches
- Calf stretch

Balance

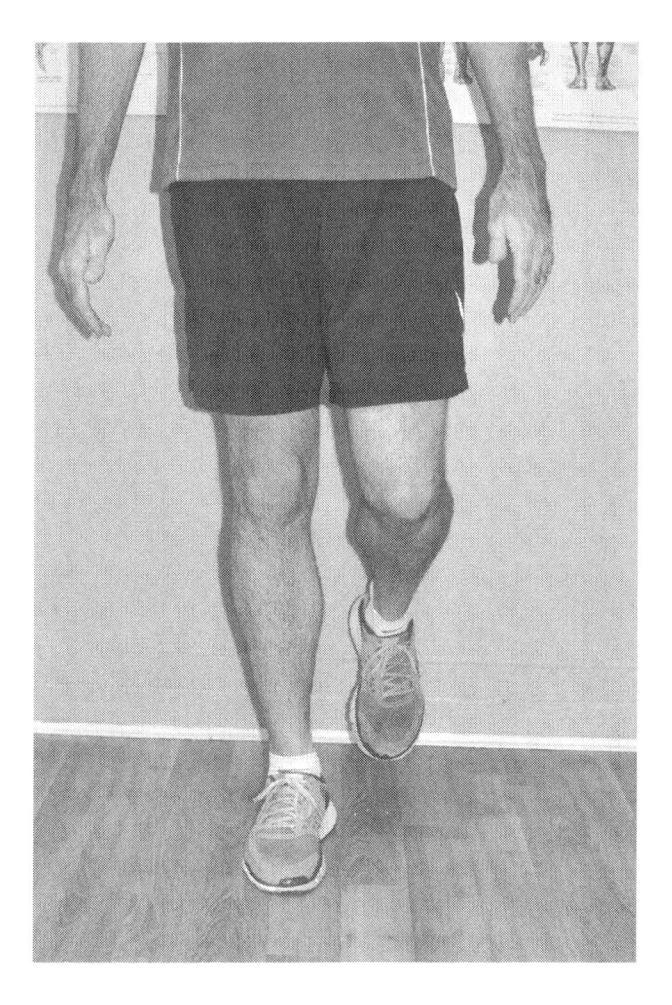

- Stand on leg - Aim for 30 seconds standing on 1 leg with your eyes open. Perform this on each leg.

Hallway exercises
1. Marching - March with high knees up and down your hallway. Swing your arms for counterbalance.
2. Side stepping - Face the wall of your hallway. Side step to your right the length of the hall. Remain facing the same wall, and side step to your left back to where you started. Make sure your hips stay facing the wall for the entire exercise.
3. Walk on toes - Lift your heels up off the ground and walk to the end of your hallway and back again on your toes.

W. 16st 1¼ 21 Feb 19.

Weeks 4 – 6

What to expect…

- **Mental Health:** Weeks 4 - 6 mark a significant change for many people. You will be feeling much better within yourself. You can truly feel the improvement now! However, don't bite off more than you can chew! Grocery shopping requires **A LOT** of walking. You are probably not ready to complete a full grocery shop yet. You will look forward to seeing your Surgeon for your Week 6 review. At this appointment, your Surgeon will allow you to return to driving. Hooray!! They will also allow you to remove your compression stockings. Hip Hip Hooray!! This is also the fortnight where you can return the over toilet frame and sit in your normal lounge chair.

- **Pain:** You will still be sore, but the level of pain will slowly be decreasing. You may still find that you are having good days and bad days. Usually, on good days, you tend to overdo things and so cause extra pain and swelling the following day. It is important that you continue to take your pain medications as directed to ensure your successful rehabilitation following surgery. You may wish to <u>begin</u> phasing out your pain medications slowly towards the end of this fortnight. Please note: stopping pain medication too soon can setback your rehabilitation by a week or more. Generally the short acting pain reliever will be the first to be reduced. However, you may still need to take these an hour prior to your physiotherapy sessions. You may also need to take one every now and then after you have overdone things. This is not a setback. It is simply a reminder to do things in moderation.

- **Swelling:** Your knee swelling will slowly reduce. You will notice that your knee swells up during the day whilst you are up and about, but reduces in size overnight as you sleep. Try to get your household tasks done in the morning, so that you can ice and elevate your legs through the afternoon. You will be getting frustrated with your compression stockings - please continue to wear them as directed!

- **Stiffness:** Your knee stiffness will continue to fluctuate. This is normal, provided you can attribute the swelling to a particular activity or to a generally busy day. For example, you spent extra time on your feet or you walked much further than usual. Continue to focus on improving your knee bend.

- **Mobility:** Your general level of mobility will continue to improve. You will find you are able to mobilise independently indoors at some point during this fortnight. You will still need one crutch outdoors throughout this fortnight. The crutch acts as a reminder to the general public to allow you greater personal space, as your balance will still be reduced. The crutch also enables you to walk further before needing a rest stop. You should practice walking quickly to eliminate any residual limp and return you to your normal gait pattern.

- **Sleep:** Your sleep should markedly improve throughout this fortnight. You may find you are now able to sleep on your side with a small pillow in between your knees to increase your comfort.

- **Physiotherapy:** Your Physiotherapist will continue to progress and expand your exercise and walking program. You may progress to fortnightly physiotherapy. Now that your scar is fully closed, you may explore hydrotherapy as an exercise option. Hydrotherapy offers you the opportunity to exercise in a warm environment that reduces both the load and impact on your knee.

- **Exercises:** Your exercise program may broaden to include exercise bike and hydrotherapy this fortnight. You will also include more balance exercises, walking drills and stretches.

- **Wound:** Your wound should be healing well and fully closed this fortnight. Many people massage moisturiser around the scar to help reduce itching and improve healing. Your Physiotherapist will be able to show your how to perform deep transverse friction massage to your scar to strengthen the scar tissue. As your scar is now fully closed, you can enter your local heated pool for Hydrotherapy (see **Physiotherapy**).

Aims for Week 6

- **Exercises** - Perform 3 x day. You will progress onto more challenging balance and weight bearing exercises.
- **Knee flexion** - Achieve 100 - 110 degrees of knee bend by Week 6.
- **Knee extension** - Achieve full knee extension - no lack or lag.
- **Mobility** - You will be walking independently indoors by Week 6. You are able to walk for 10 - 20 minutes on flat ground outside with no difficulties. You may still need 1 crutch outside at Week 6.

Risks & Complications

The main complications at this time are:
- Blood clots – You can stop wearing your compression stockings at 6 weeks.

- Infection – Your wound should now be fully closed. However, infection can travel from other parts of your body (such as a scratch on your arm) to your new knee, so please continue to monitor for signs of infection.

- Stiffness - Your knee will stiffen up if you overdo your walking and exercises. This is not a race! Perform your rehabilitation at a moderate pace and you will enjoy a full recovery. You will now start to see rapid improvement this fortnight and feel much more comfortable with your progress. You may slowly reduce the amount of pain relief you are taking (as appropriate) and may reduce your physiotherapy visits to fortnightly. You will have good days and bad days. You will tend to overdo things on the good days and then suffer for this the following day. Don't be concerned by this, just be aware and try to moderate your activities.

Exercise Program - Week 5

Circulatory exercises - Perform these only if your leg swelling is persistent.
- Buttock squeezes
- Thigh squeezes
- Ankle pumps

Bed exercises - Continue to perform these 3 x day.
- Thigh squeezes
- Inner range quads
- Straight leg raise
- Passive knee extension over roll
- Heel slides

Seated Exercises - Continue to perform these 3 x day.
- Seated knee extension
- Seated knee bend with skateboard.
- Sit to stand
- Scar massage

Position: Seated with leg elevated on a stool. Knee is relaxed.

Action: Place your thumb on the top end of the healed scar and press downward to sink to your deeper skin layers. Holding this position, move your thumb towards the inside of your thigh, and then towards the outside of your thigh. Repeat this movement for about 5 seconds and then move one thumb's width downward along the scar and repeat the massage.

Repeat: All the way along the length of your scar provided it has fully closed over. Avoid any areas where the scar has not completely healed.

Frequency: 3 x day

Walking - You should be walking for roughly 15 minutes per day outside. You may still require 1 crutch this week.

Stairs - Continue to practice these daily if you have them at home.

Bench exercises - Continue to perform these 3 x day.
- Calf raises
- Swing leg out to the side
- March on spot
- Kick butt
- Shallow squat
- **Lunges -** This combines the strengthening of a squat whilst challenging your balance.

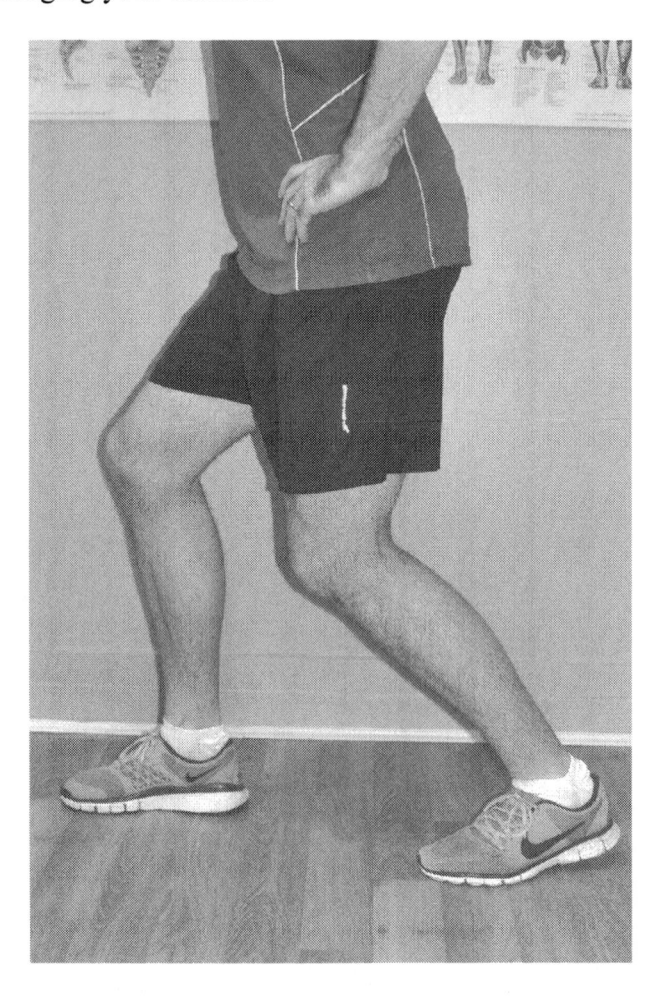

Position: Stand with feet together alongside a bench or chair.
Action: Step forward, allowing your front knee to bend as you shift your body weight forward. Ensure that as your knee bends, it remains square over your front foot. Your back leg remains fixed. Your heel can rise up off the ground if that is more comfortable. Step back so that your feet are together once more.
Repeat: Alternate legs and perform 20 in total (10 per leg)
Frequency: 3 x day.
Note: You can adjust the amount of body weight through your front leg if you find the lunges are a bit to challenging.

Stretches
- Calf stretch

Balance
- **Stand on leg** - Aim for 30 seconds standing on 1 leg with your eyes open. Perform this on each leg.
- **Heel-toe** - Pretend you are walking along a tightrope, placing the heel of one foot directly in front of the toes of the other foot. Do this up and down your hallway.

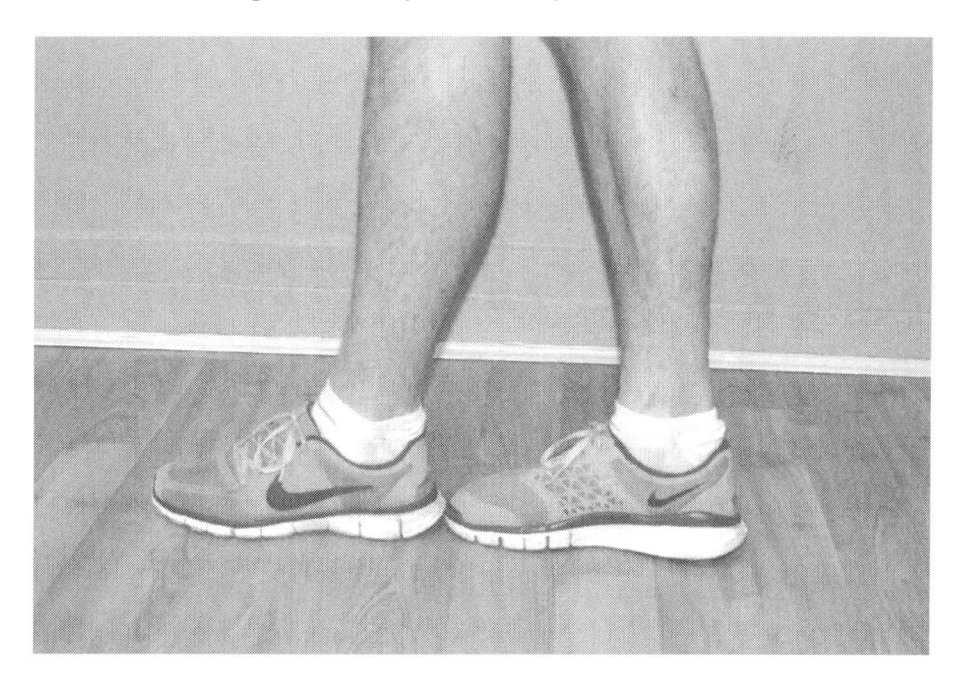

Hallway exercises
1. Marching
2. Side stepping
3. Walk on toes
4. **Walk backwards** - Make sure there are no hazards such as rugs, cords, hallway tables in the way! Walk backwards up and down your hallway. If you don't feel safe, do this when you have your support person present, or do this alongside your kitchen bench.

Exercise Program - Week 6

Bed exercises - Continue to perform these 3 x day.
- Thigh squeezes
- Inner range quads
- Straight leg raise
- Passive knee extension over roll
- Heel slides

Seated Exercises - Continue to perform these 3 x day.
- Seated knee extension
- Seated knee bend with skateboard.
- Sit to stand
- Scar massage

Walking - You should be walking for roughly 20 minutes per day outside. You should be independent this week.

Stairs - Continue to practice these daily if you have them at home.

Bench exercises - Continue to perform these 3 x day.
- Calf raises
- Swing leg out to the side
- March on spot
- Kick butt
- Shallow squat
- Lunges

Stretches
- Calf stretch

○ **Hamstring stretch -**

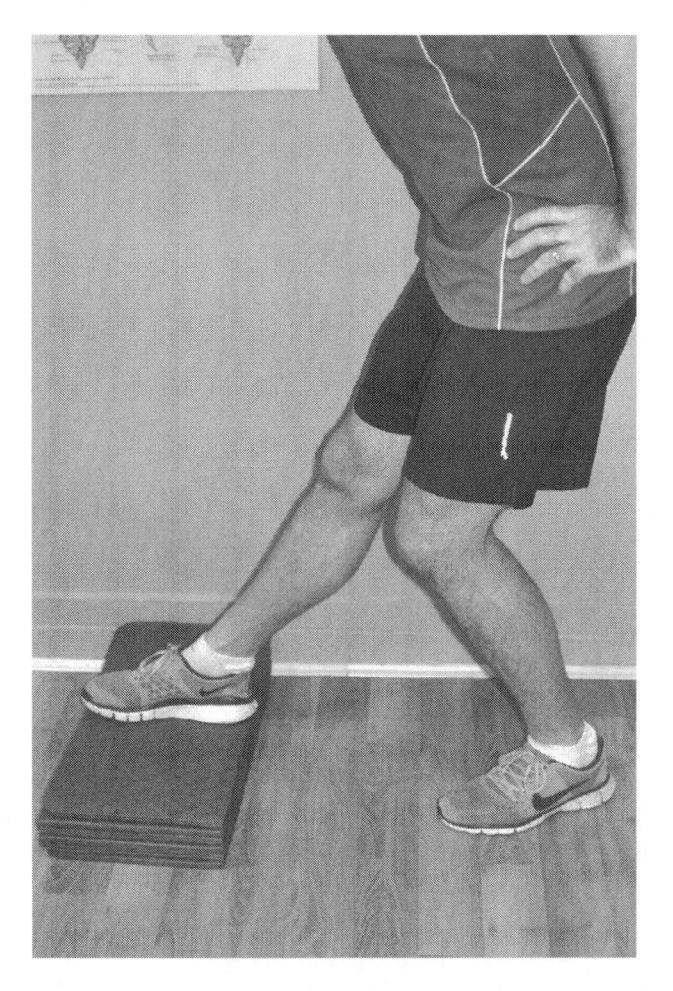

Position: Position a foot stool next to the kitchen bench.
Action: Place the foot of a straight leg onto the stool. Keep your knee straight. Gently lean forward from your hips and feel a stretch in the muscle behind your thigh (hamstring muscle).
Repeat: Hold the stretch for 30 seconds. Perform once on each leg.
Frequency: 3 x day.
Note: Avoid rotating your leg by ensuring that your foot is pointing straight up to the ceiling.

Balance
- Stand on leg - As you achieve 30 seconds with your eyes open, try performing this with your eyes closed and feel the difference!
- Heel-toe

Hallway exercises
- Marching
- Side stepping
- Walk on toes
- Walk backwards
- **Walking lunges -**

Position: Perform these down your hallway. Think 1 - 2 - 3...Step - down - up.

Action: Take a step forward, perform a lunge, step forward onto the next foot. Repeat.

Repeat: Down the length of your hallway.

Frequency: 3 x day.

Note: Don't rush these!

Exercise bike - If you have access to an exercise bike, this week is a good time to start using it. Ensure that you position the seat higher than normal and you do not have any resistance to pedalling. Begin with 5 minutes of pedalling, once daily for this week. If you overdo it on the bike, you can cause your knee to swell.

Weeks 6 – 8

What to expect...

- **Mental Health:** Weeks 6 - 8 can be a risky period for those patients who tend to overdo things. Those patients who have pushed too hard in the first 6 weeks may find that they have overstepped, and their knee can suddenly swell and stiffen this fortnight. This is why it is so important that you follow your exercise program in moderation. You may have returned to work, but this varies greatly depending on the nature of your work. Those in sedentary, office based work may find they can return this fortnight. Just remember that you will have lost a great deal of work fitness and may find you are more fatigued than you expected by the end of the week.

- **Pain:** You should now have weaned off the fast acting pain reliever and be in the process of weaning off your slow release pain reliever. By Week 8 you should be only taking paracetamol as required.

- **Swelling:** Your knee may feel warm or appear slightly different to your other knee. This is completely normal. There will be a degree of warmth and swelling for a few months. You won't be needing regular ice anymore.

- **Stiffness:** Your knee should be moving quite well at this point. It may still stiffen from time to time depending on your level of recent activity, but this stiffening will become less and less frequent.

- **Mobility:** Your gait pattern should have returned to normal by Week 8.

- **Sleep:** Your sleep should have returned to normal by Week 8. You can sleep on your back or either side quite well. Those who sleep on their stomachs may still find it a bit uncomfortable, but this varies patient to patient.

- **Physiotherapy:** Your Physiotherapist will continue to progress and expand your exercise and walking program. You may progress to fortnightly physiotherapy. Now that your scar is fully closed, you may explore hydrotherapy as a therapy option. Hydrotherapy offers you the opportunity to exercise in a warm environment that reduces both the load and impact on your knee.

- **Exercises:** You will continue to perform the more challenging exercises 3 x day up until Week 8.

- **Wound:** Your scar is becoming thinner, flatter and lighter in colour. It should now be quite mobile and no longer feel like it is sticking to any deeper structures in your knee when you massage it.

Aims for Week 8

- **Exercises** - Perform 3 x day. Continue your more challenging balance and weight bearing exercises.
- **Knee flexion** - Achieve 115 - 120 degrees of knee bend by Week 8. This will vary patient to patient.
- **Knee extension** - Achieve full knee extension - no lack or lag.
- **Mobility** - You will be walking independently indoors and outdoors by Week 8. You are able to walk for 30 minutes on flat ground outside with no difficulties.

Risks & Complications

The main complications at this time are:
- Stiffness - Your knee will stiffen up if you overdo your walking and exercises. This is not a race! Perform your rehabilitation at a moderate pace and you will enjoy a full recovery. You will

now start to see rapid improvement this fortnight and feel much more comfortable with your progress. You may slowly reduce the amount of pain relief you are taking (as appropriate) and may reduce your physiotherapy visits to fortnightly. You will have good days and bad days. You will tend to overdo things on the good days and then suffer for this the following day. Don't be concerned by this, just be aware and try to moderate your activities. You can really start to get out and about again. But this increase in activity can result in an increase in pain, swelling and stiffness and you may feel like it is a setback. As long as you can attribute those symptoms to an increased activity level, don't be concerned. Just monitor your knee and adjust your activities accordingly.

Exercise Program - Week 6 - 8

Bed exercises - Continue to perform these 3 x day.
- Inner range quads
- Straight leg raise
- Heel slides

Seated Exercises - Continue to perform these 3 x day.
- Seated knee extension
- Seated knee bend with skateboard.
- Scar massage

Walking - You should be walking independently for 30 minutes per day outside by the end of Week 8.

Stairs - Continue to practice these daily if you have them at home.

Bench exercises - Continue to perform these 3 x day.
- Calf raises
- Swing leg out to the side
- March on spot
- Kick butt
- Shallow squat
- Lunges

Stretches
- Calf stretch
- Hamstring stretch

o **Lower back/buttock stretch -**

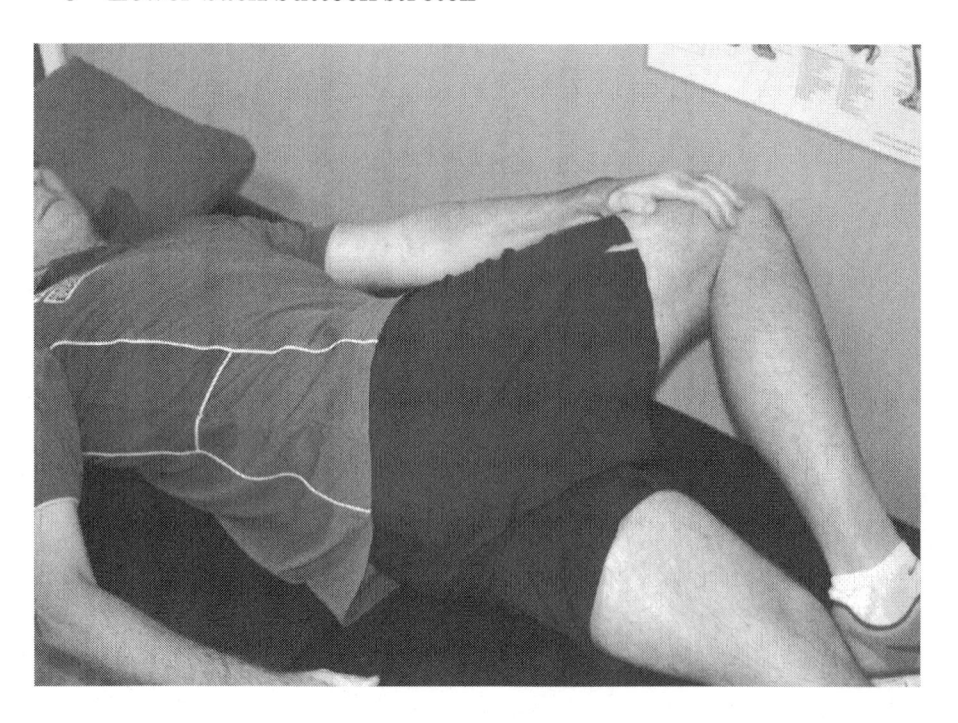

Position: Lay face up on your bed, with your knee bent and your feet flat on the bed.
Action: Keeping your knees together, rotate them slowly towards the bed on your left. Straighten out your bottom leg. Use your left hand to apply downward pressure to your top knee to feel an extra stretch through your buttocks. Hold the stretch for 10 seconds, then slowly rotate them over to the right side. Repeat the downward pressure with your right hand and hold for a further 10 seconds.
Repeat: Once per side.
Frequency: Daily.

- **Lower back stretch -**

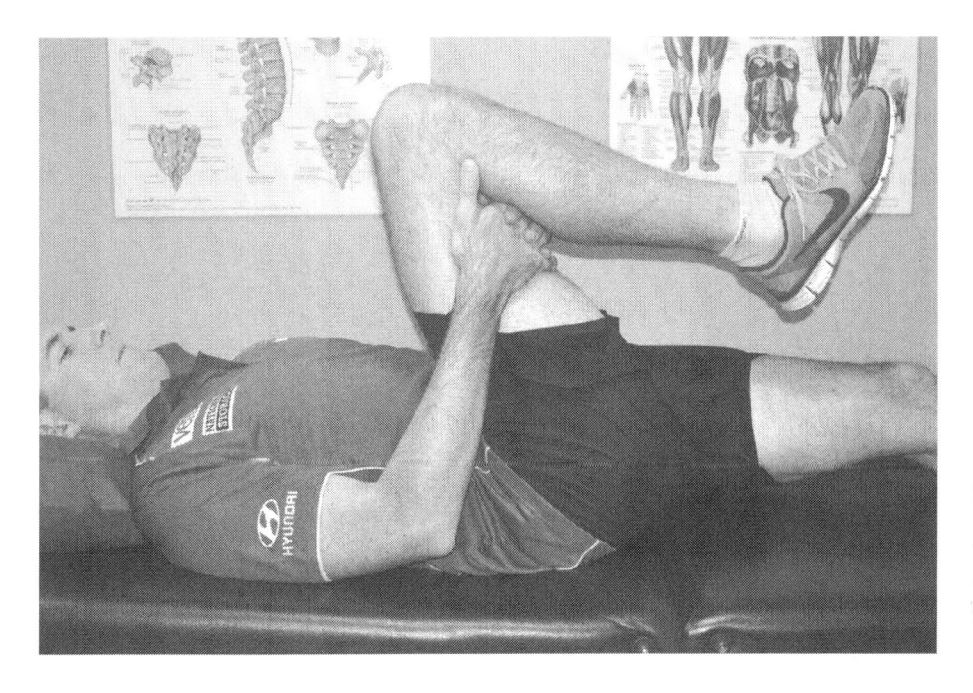

Position: Lay face up on your bed.
Action: Grasp around the end of your thigh. Gently pull your thigh towards your chest. Your foot will be in the air. You should feel a gentle stretch in your lower back.
Repeat: Hold for 10 seconds, then repeat on the other side.
Frequency: Daily.

Balance
- Stand on leg - Eyes open, eyes closed or try on an uneven surface such as grass, sand, or a folded towel on the floor.
- Heel-toe - Try this walking both forwards and also backwards.

Hallway exercises
- Marching
- Side stepping
- Walk on toes
- Walk backwards
- Walking lunges

- **Walking on heels** - Lift your toes up off the ground and walk up and down your hallway on your heels.

Exercise bike - Gradually increase your time on the bike by 5 minutes each week. You should make 15 minutes by the end of week 8. You can also try to slowly lower the seat to gradually increase the maximal amount of knee bend which occurs at the top of each cycle.

Hydrotherapy - Now that your wound is completely healed, you can consider exercising in a hydrotherapy pool. See the Hydrotherapy section for a complete program. Limit your sessions to 20 minutes at a time.

Weeks 8 – 12

What to expect...

- **Mental Health:** You will be feeling more confident and be returning to most of your regular activities. You will be looking forward to your 12 week review with your surgeon. You will have an x-ray of your knee to check the status of your prosthesis.

- **Pain:** You should no longer be requiring regular pain relief. You may still feel occasional knee soreness that may or may not require pain relief.

- **Swelling:** Your knee may feel warm or appear slightly different to your other knee. This is completely normal. There will be a degree of warmth and swelling for a few months. You won't be needing regular ice anymore.

- **Stiffness:** Your knee should be moving freely by Week 12. You may have occasional stiffness in your knee related to a larger than usual amount of exercise.

- **Mobility:** You should be walking regularly and with a normal gait pattern.

- **Sleep:** You should have returned to your regular sleep patterns. Those who sleep on their stomachs may still find it a bit uncomfortable, but this varies patient to patient.

- **Physiotherapy:** You will probably have your final physiotherapy session sometime this month. Now it's up to you to continue your exercises until you achieve your personal goals.

- **Exercises:** You can reduce your exercises to 2 x day until Week 10. Then once daily until Week 12.

- **Wound:** Your scar is becoming thinner, flatter and lighter in colour. It should now be quite mobile and no longer feel like it is sticking to any deeper structures in your knee when you massage it.

Aims for Week 12

- **Exercises** - Perform 2 x day from Week 8 - 10. Then daily from Week 10 - 12.
- **Knee flexion** - up to 130 - 140 degrees
- **Knee extension** - Full
- **Mobility** - You will be returning to your regular activities. You are able to walk for 45 - 60 minutes on flat ground outside by Week 12.

Risks & Complications

The main complications at this time are:

- Stiffness - If stiffness is persisting through Weeks 8 - 12 without marked improvement, you will need to discuss with your options with your surgeon. In particular, whether a manipulation under anaesthesia is required.

- Intermittent pain - As you extend your activities and perhaps return to work, you may find that you suffer from intermittent knee pain and even intermittent swelling. This is normal, provided you can attribute this to increased activity.

Exercise Program - Week 8 - 10

Bed exercises - Perform these 2 x day.
- Inner range quads
- Straight leg raise

Seated Exercises - Perform these 2 x day.
- Seated knee extension
- Seated knee bend with skateboard.

Walking - You should be walking independently for 30 - 40 minutes per day outside by the end of Week 10.

Stairs - Continue to practice these daily if you have them at home.

Bench exercises - Perform these 2 x day.
- Calf raises
- Swing leg out to the side
- March on spot
- Kick butt
- Shallow squat
- Lunges

Stretches - Perform these 2 x day
- Calf stretch
- Hamstring stretch
- Lower back/buttock stretch
- Lower back stretch

Balance - Perform these 2 x day
- Stand on leg
- Heel-toe

Hallway exercises - Perform these 2 x day
- Marching

- Side stepping
- Walk on toes
- Walk backwards
- Walking lunges
- Walk on heels

Exercise bike - You should be able to achieve 25 - 30 minutes on the exercise bike. This can replace an outdoors walk. You may like to use the exercise bike one day, and then go for a long walk the following day.

Hydrotherapy - Use this as an alternative to one of your daily exercise sessions. You can increase your session length to 30 minutes.

Exercise Program - Week 10 - 12

Bed exercises - Perform these daily.
- Straight leg raise

Seated Exercises - Perform these daily.
- Seated knee bend with skateboard.

Walking - You should be walking independently for 45 - 60 minutes per day outside by the end of Week 12.

Stairs - Continue to practice these daily if you have them at home.

Bench exercises - Perform these daily.
- Calf raises
- Kick butt
- Shallow squat
- Lunges

Stretches - Perform these daily.
- Calf stretch
- Hamstring stretch
- Lower back/buttock stretch
- Lower back stretch

Balance - Perform these daily.
- Stand on leg
- Heel-toe

Hallway exercises - Perform these daily.
- Marching
- Side stepping
- Walk on toes
- Walk backwards
- Walking lunges

- Walk on heels

Exercise bike - 30 minutes on the exercise bike. This can replace an outdoors walk. You may like to use the exercise bike one day, and then go for a long walk the following day. You can increase the resistance, or lower the seat for extra challenge.

Hydrotherapy - Use this as an alternative to one of your daily exercise sessions. You can extend your session to 30 - 40 minutes long.

Week 12 and beyond...

How you approach weeks 12 and beyond really depends on your personal goals and whether you wish/need to return to work/sport etc. Unless there have been complications due to adhesions, excessive pain or swelling, you should no longer be requiring regular physiotherapy. You will have seen your surgeon for your 12 week review. They will probably want to see you in 6 months time, then yearly up until 5 years post-surgery. During that time it is important to continue doing the more challenging exercises 2 – 3 times per week. I have included an exercise plan below this section with the more challenging exercises you should consider. If you are returning to work or sport, you should also be practising exercises or drills that are specific to your work/sport needs. These will vary quite dramatically depending on your type of work or sport, so are not covered specifically in this book. You should consider all aspects of your work/sport and practise each component until you feel confident to return safely.

Niggles
You may encounter the niggles listed below in the time after week 12.

Heat
Your knee may feel warm for months. This is normal as your prosthesis is a foreign object and your body is still getting used to it. Unless there is a rapid increase in knee temperature, don't worry. Call your doctor if you have any concerns.

Occasional swelling/soreness/stiffness/tightness
This will occur if you have overdone things. Often it is not one activity, but the cumulative effect of many little things that adds up over the day or across the week. It will be a sign that you need to take it easy for a few days before getting back into the swing of things again. You can use ice, self-massage, over the counter pain relief and gentle exercises to help relieve these symptoms.

Kneeling
Many people find kneeling uncomfortable after having a knee replacement. Don't be concerned if you can't kneel just yet. It may be

helpful to try kneeling on your bed at first, as it is well cushioned and is easier to get up afterward. Once you are confident, try kneeling on a thick cushion on the floor, then progress onto soft surfaces such as thick carpet or grass, before eventually trying a harder floor. This can take months to achieve for some people, so there is no need to rush. Just do what feels comfortable for you at the time.

Other joints
Remember - arthritis is often not limited to one joint. You may find now that the "worst joint" has been fixed, the second worst joint may now feel quite sore and you will wonder where this has come from. Also, the stronger leg has had to carry you for the past few months, let alone the previous months/years prior to surgery. It may now be sore. If rest, over the counter pain relief, gentle exercise and gentle heat do not relieve or manage your symptoms, you may need to see your doctor to discuss the need for an x-ray to review the status of this new sore area.

Podiatrist
You may find now that your knees have been straightened, you notice that one leg seems longer than the other, or that your ankle seems to roll inward/outward more than it did prior to surgery. If this concerns you, I recommend you see your local podiatrist once you are 12 weeks post-surgery. They will assess your feet and posture and determine whether you require an orthotic or other adjustment for your shoes.

Exercise Program - Week 12 and Beyond...

As an ongoing exercise program, you should continue the exercises listed below 2 - 3 times per week to keep your knee in top condition.

Bed exercises
- Straight leg raise

Walking - up to 50 - 60 minutes if able. Gentle slopes are now permitted.

Stairs

Bench exercises
- Calf raises
- Kick butt
- Shallow squat
- Lunges

Stretches
- Calf stretch
- Hamstring stretch
- Lower back/buttock stretch
- Lower back stretch

Balance
- Stand on leg
- Heel-toe

Hallway exercises
- Marching
- Side stepping
- Walk on toes
- Walk backwards
- Walking lunges
- Walk on heels

Exercise bike - 30 minutes on the exercise bike. This can replace an outdoors walk. You can increase the resistance, or lower the seat for extra challenge.

Hydrotherapy - Use this as an alternative to one of your daily exercise sessions. You can extend your session to 30 - 40 minutes long.

It's up to you…

Congratulations!

You've made it to 12 weeks after your knee replacement and you should be feeling proud of yourself.

As you move forward I just want to remind you of a few key points:

- Keep up the more challenging exercises 2 - 3 times per week for good. Your knees will thank you.
- Eat a nutritious diet and be as active and strong as you can. This will help with weight control and reduce the stresses on your knees.
- You may still have good and bad days for the next few months. As long as you can attribute this to increased activity, don't be concerned. Simply ensure you have a few quiet days scheduled after any hectic period.
- As always, if you have any concerns, speak with your family doctor or your surgeon. It's better to be safe than sorry.

If you have found Total Knee Replacement - 12 Weeks to Success helpful, please leave a review on Amazon.

If you would like a free 12 Week Exercise Planner to help keep track of your exercises, visit www.thetotalkneereplacement.com and enter your name and email address and you will receive a printable PDF in your in-box.

Thank you for reading Total Knee Replacement - 12 Weeks to Success. I wish you all the very best for a complete and speedy recovery.

LORI MARSHALL

Glossary

Active Range of Movement
The amount of movement at a joint when you move voluntarily, using your own muscle strength. It is measured in degrees.

Adhesions
Thick, heavy scar tissue that can limit the amount of movement of your knee. A small amount can be remedied by physiotherapy, but larger adhesions require a manipulation under anaesthesia to restore full range of motion to the joint.

Bilateral Knee Replacement
Undergoing both left and right knee replacements in a single surgical procedure.

Calf
The muscle that allows you to lift your heels up off the ground and stand on your toes. It sits behind your shin bone.

Continuous Passive Motion Machine
A machine that your surgeon may choose to use whilst you are in hospital, or after you have had a manipulation under anaesthesia. Your leg is positioned on the machine and your knee is repeatedly flexed and extended to slowly improve your range of motion and limit the formation of adhesions.

Extension
The straightening of your knee as you move your heel away from your bottom.

Flexion
The bending of your knee as you move your heel towards your bottom.

Hamstrings
The muscle that bends your knee. It sits behind your thigh.

Lack
How far from full extension your knee is when your Physiotherapist or Surgeon straighten your knee. It is measured in degrees.

Lag
How far from full extension your knee is when you straighten it voluntarily using your muscle strength. It is measured in degrees.

Manipulation Under Anaesthesia
A non-surgical procedure where you are placed under either general or spinal anaesthesia to enable your surgeon to manipulate your knee without causing you pain or muscle spasm to break any adhesions that are restricting your range of motion.

Passive Range of Movement
The amount of movement at a joint when it is moved without effort from you, such as when your Surgeon or Physiotherapist moves your knee. It is measured in degrees.

Prosthesis
An artificial device that replaces your knee joint. It can be made from metal or hard plastic.

Quadriceps
The muscle that straightens your knee. It has four parts to the muscle and is situated on the front of your thigh. It is also known as the "Quads".

Total Knee Replacement or Knee Arthroplasty
A Total Knee Replacement is a major surgical procedure, where the damaged areas of the knee joint are replaced with a metal and plastic artificial knee joint. It is also known as a "Knee Arthroplasty".

Bibliography

American Association of Orthopedic Surgeons, 2015, *Total Knee Replacement*, www.orthoinfo.com.

Australian Orthopaedic Association, New Zealand Orthopaedic Association, 2014, *Surgical Replacement of the Knee Joint - A Guide for Patients,* www.mitec.com.au.

Dekkers, Dr M, 2016, *Guide to Expectations Following A Computer Navigated Total Knee Replacement.*

Greenslopes Private Hospital, 2013, *Care of you and your new knee,* Ramsay Healthcare.

Self Care Therapy, 2016, *How to put on Compression Stockings*, www.selfcaretherapy.com.

ABOUT THE AUTHOR

Lori Marshall has rehabilitated hundreds of patients after Total Knee Replacement surgery in Brisbane, Australia. After graduating as a Physiotherapist from the University of Queensland in 2002, she worked in Aged Care and Private Practice settings, before establishing her in-home physiotherapy service.

In between massaging legs and bending knees, Lori enjoys playing on the wing of her touch football team with her husband, Evan, and kicking a soccer ball at the park with her two sons, Charlie and Henry. She hopes that keeping fit will help her avoid a knee replacement in the future.

Printed in Great Britain
by Amazon